Praise for *The Vitamin D Revolution*

"Did you know that there is an epidemic of vitamin D deficiency in America? Did you know that a lack of proper vitamin D has been scientifically connected to 17 varieties of cancer, along with many other life-threatening diseases? Did you know that vitamin D isn't even a vitamin (it's a hormone)? You will after reading this practical and information-packed guide to a powerful (yet inexpensive) 'wonder vitamin' that can markedly improve your health. I've experienced firsthand that Dr. Soram is riding the wave of the medical future— focused on prevention, and combining the best of traditional Western medicine with alternative approaches."

— **Arianna Huffington**, nationally syndicated columnist

"Smart . . . smart . . . smart! Dr. Khalsa is one of America's top integrative medicine doctors. In his impeccably researched book, he offers important new advice that can help make your children and family healthier . . . and could even save your life!"

— **Harvey Karp, M.D., FAAP,** creator of the book and DVD, *The Happiest Baby on the Block*

"I would pull my chair up and listen very closely to anything Dr. Soram Khalsa says; he is one of the most brilliant, well-researched, and intuitive doctors I have ever met. Always three steps ahead of everyone else, Khalsa is a wise sage who will lead us into our ultimate health."

— **Kathy Freston**, the *New York Times* best-selling author of *Quantum Wellness*

"The Vitamin D Revolution is a wonderful and very timely book for the African-American community on becoming aware of the importance of vitamin D. As a patient of Dr. Khalsa, I truly experience the ultimate health and recommend this book to everyone."

— **Verdine White**, co-founder of the Grammy Award–winning band Earth, Wind & Fire

"Dr. Khalsa has written an easy to understand summary of the current literature on vitamin D. He has nicely pointed out that we are experiencing an epidemic of vitamin D deficiency, in great part due to the use of sunscreen, protective clothing, and avoidance of sun exposure. Since vitamin D deficiency is associated with osteoporosis and other medical problems, and since it is so easily diagnosed and corrected, Dr. Khalsa is performing a public service by increasing the awareness of this problem. He has appropriately pointed out that studies that show an association between low vitamin D levels and disease states do not necessarily indicate that the disease is due to the vitamin D deficiency. Nevertheless, he provides a reasonable argument that correcting a low vitamin D level is a good thing to do, since there is very little downside, as long as one does not take massive doses of the vitamin. He advocates measurement of blood vitamin D levels to diagnose deficiency and to monitor therapy. I applaud Dr. Khalsa's strong advocacy for this important health issue."*

— **Glenn D. Braunstein, M.D.**, Chairman, Department of Medicine, Cedars-Sinai Medical Center, Los Angeles, California

"This book simplifies vitamin D research on 20+ diseases, and provides practical guidelines for patients and physicians concerning finding optimal levels of vitamin D intake and serum targets for 25-hydroxyvitamin D. You'll enjoy reading it if you're interested in preventive medicine and your personal health."

— **Cedric F. Garland, Dr. P.H., F.A.C.E.**, adjunct professor of Family and Preventive Medicine, University of California, San Diego, Moores Cancer Center; widely published vitamin D researcher

the
VITAMIN D
REVOLUTION

Hay House Titles of Related Interest

the VITAMIN D REVOLUTION

How the Power of This Amazing Vitamin Can Change Your Life

Soram Khalsa, M.D.

HAY HOUSE, INC.
Carlsbad, California • New York City
London • Sydney • Johannesburg
Vancouver • Hong Kong • New Delhi

Copyright © 2009 by Soram Khalsa

Published and distributed in the United States by: Hay House, Inc.: www.hayhouse
.com • *Published and distributed in Australia by:* Hay House Australia Pty. Ltd.: www
.hayhouse.com.au • *Published and distributed in the United Kingdom by:* Hay House
UK, Ltd.: www.hayhouse.co.uk • *Published and distributed in the Republic of South
Africa by:* Hay House SA (Pty), Ltd.: www.hayhouse.co.za • *Distributed in Canada by:*
Raincoast: www.raincoast.com • *Published in India by:* Hay House Publishers India:
www.hayhouse.co.in

Editorial supervision: Jill Kramer • *Design:* Nick C. Welch
Interior illustrations courtesy of the author

Throughout this book, all patient names have been changed.

Library of Congress Cataloging-in-Publication Data

Khalsa, Soram.
  The vitamin D revolution : how the power of this amazing vitamin can change your life / Soram Khalsa.
    p. cm.
  Includes bibliographical references.
  ISBN 978-1-4019-2470-6 (tradepaper : alk. paper) 1. Vitamin D--Popular works. 2. Vitamin D in human nutrition--Popular works. I. Title.
  QP772.V53K53 2009
  612.3'99--dc22

                                    2008047704

ISBN: 978-1-4019-2470-6

13 12 11 10   5 4 3 2
1st edition, March 2009
2nd edition, February 2010

Printed By CPI Bookmarque, Croydon

*To Yogi Bhajan, my spiritual teacher,
who guided me to be who and what I am.*

CONTENTS

Preface

THE VITAMIN D REVOLUTION

There is a revolution that is about to take place in medicine. It began quietly more than ten years ago in hidden-away research labs. However, in the six months prior to writing this book, awareness of this phenomenon has begun to reach every newspaper, magazine, and Website in the world. I predict that it will not be long until everyone on Earth feels and understands the power of this revolution and how it can change the world.

This revolution is the result of new research on the power that vitamin D offers us to improve human health and longevity. Vitamin D deficiency is now connected with 17 varieties of cancer, along with heart disease, high blood pressure, strokes, autoimmune diseases, diabetes, chronic pain, and osteoporosis. Initially, these research studies have shown that there is a strong relationship between vitamin D and these diseases. But now the studies are shifting to more comprehensive so-called randomized-controlled trials (RCT), the gold standard of medical studies, and I predict that these will transform the way medicine is practiced.

We are no longer at the beginning of understanding the power of vitamin D. I believe that with the strength of all the studies we already have, combined with the new ones coming out, there is sufficient evidence for a mandate to the government to raise the RDA (recommended daily allowance) for vitamin D. Everyone should be tested (just as they are for diabetes and cholesterol); and all physicians, regardless of their area of specialization, should stand up and normalize their patients' levels of this amazingly powerful vitamin-hormone.

◻◼◻

While practicing medicine as a board-certified internist with a special focus in integrative medicine for more than 30 years, I have seen many medical trends.

In the 1970s, everybody had hypoglycemia. In the 1980s, it was chronic fatigue syndrome, and in the 1990s, everybody had fibromyalgia. All of these diagnoses are real, and even now I treat many patients with these conditions. However, over this entire time, I have never seen any medical diagnosis as widespread and so profoundly affecting people's health and well-being as the current epidemic of vitamin D deficiency.

I first became aware of the pivotal role that vitamin D plays in human health over five years ago. It was while listening to my colleague and friend Dr. Jeffrey Bland's monthly audio CDs that I heard of the importance of vitamin D for the immune system.

Shortly thereafter, at an Institute for Functional Medicine colloquium, I listened to a lecture by Michael Holick, M.D., Ph.D., from Boston University. His talk began with a dramatic video of a rising sun with the music of *Thus Spake Zarathustra* playing loudly. Chills ran through my spine, and I knew I was in for a treat. This was not like any lecture I had ever attended.

Dr. Holick then went on to explain the ubiquitous appearance of vitamin D in almost every tissue in the human body. He explained that what we had thought was a vitamin was subsequently shown to be a hormone—not a vitamin. In addition, he also explained how it was linked to so many diseases throughout the entire body.

Dr. Holick revealed the fact that the current dosages recommended as the RDA for vitamin D were simply based upon outdated research on preventing rickets and needed to be updated to our current understanding of it. He also explained why the normal blood range of vitamin D that we were taught in medical school— anything above 20 nanograms per milliliter (ng/ml)— was not nearly enough, according to the ongoing current research.

I went home from that lecture and began to read everything I could find on vitamin D in medical journals and books. I attended more lectures on vitamin D, and my understanding and appreciation of the power of this so-called vitamin deepened. I also measured my own level and found myself—with my fair skin and my Sikh clothing, which covered almost all of me—to be woefully depleted of vitamin D.

I then began to measure my patients. Here I am in Los Angeles (most recently, Beverly Hills), the "Land of the Sun," and I had guessed that all of my patients, who do not wear the type of protective clothing I do, would have normal levels. Wow! Was I wrong! Since that time, I have continued to measure vitamin D levels in every new patient as well as in my current patients as part of their annual physicals. In my practice, I have found that over 75 percent of all my new patients have insufficient levels.

Because the sun is our major source of vitamin D and we have so much of it in Southern California, I had assumed that people would be getting their vitamin D from the sun. But then I remembered that most of my patients see their dermatologists regularly, and that for many years they have been warning all of us about the dangers of sun exposure and its role in creating skin cancer. They have trained us to shield ourselves before we even go out for the day. Indeed, most women's cosmetics now have some sun protection in them. I realized that so many of my patients were testing low in their vitamin D levels because they were all using sunblock.

I acknowledged that we must create a new relationship with the sun. Depending on which of the six skin types we as individuals have, it is important for us to get some sunshine on a regular basis. (You will learn much more about this as you read on.) In addition, I realized that it was critical to do a blood test in order to measure my patients' blood levels of vitamin D. Those who were low could then be given a large dose for a relatively short time to bring them up to normal, and thereafter be kept on a maintenance dose.

I have been doing this actively in my practice now for more than five years, and I have witnessed many miracles unfold just by normalizing an individual's vitamin D level. I will talk more about this later.

Awhile ago, I came across an advertisement for finger-stick vitamin D blood measurements from a laboratory that I had been working closely with for other tests. These were "stick yourself at home" tests that patients could send directly to a lab. Because we draw blood all the time at my office, I did not think much of this.

Then during my meditation one day, the thought came to me that a home test would be perfect for the millions of patients who do not see a doctor regularly or whose doctors are not performing vitamin D blood tests regularly. I also realized that I could provide these test kits to people at a very reasonable price. But then I asked myself, *How will patients know what to do with their test results?*

That is when it became imperative that I write this book. I knew it had to be written in lay language and be simple and to the point, as well as being an enjoyable and quick read. In a book, I could teach readers how I correct my patients' vitamin D levels and bring them up to either normal or optimal range, depending on their particular health picture or personal needs. Allowing people to have access to a test kit would enable them to take control of their own health and ascertain their vitamin D status. And then from this book, they could learn the dosages I advise for my patients so that they could achieve normal and optimal levels. Of course, the other good thing about the test kits is that after a period of time, people can repeat their tests and keep tabs on their progress.

Then came the problem of obtaining quality vitamin D capsules. A recent report in the medical literature, published by Dr. Holick, stated that one patient bought vitamin D capsules from a health-food store that had been significantly mislabeled. Indeed, the actual amount in these particular pills was approximately 100 times what was on the label!

Because vitamin D in excess amounts can lead to toxicity, this patient developed toxic symptoms and required hospitalization, although he subsequently recovered from his vitamin D toxicity. This is one reason why measuring your own level is so critical—not only can you bring yourself up to an optimal level, but you can do so without overdosing.

However, I do want you to know that overdosing to the point of toxicity is very hard to do. Over these last years, several of my patients have taken a higher dose than I advised, and although their levels went into the high-normal range, none of them has ever become toxic.

Because of this problem with the possible unreliability of health-food store vitamin D, I contacted a nutritional supplement company that only supplies products to health professionals. This company conducts extremely careful quality control, follows "Good Manufacturing Practices" (regulations enforced by the FDA), and has in-house laboratory scientists measuring every batch and confirming the dose with a "Certificate of Analysis." They have agreed to partner with me to provide high-quality, reasonably priced, guaranteed-dosage vitamin D supplements so that the readers of this book can be certain that the dosage they are receiving will be accurate.

I am very excited about the possibility of improving the health of our country, and indeed the entire world, by helping every person to safely achieve normal or—even better—optimal vitamin D levels. It is my sincere belief that all the benefits of this "vitamin-hormone" will improve their quality of life and extend their years of healthy living.

I look forward to taking you along with me on this vitamin D adventure! I hope that you will become as excited about this inexpensive, easy-to-obtain "vitamin" as I am.

— **Soram Khalsa**, M.D.
Beverly Hills, California

■■■ ■■■

Introduction

WHAT'S IN THIS BOOK

Chapter One: How Our Understanding of Vitamin D Has Evolved

In Chapter 1, I explain how our scientific understanding of vitamin D has evolved from being a simple substance necessary for bone health into an essential nutrient whose optimal usage reduces mortality rates. Of particular importance is some information about the origins of the public's fear of vitamin D toxicity. I clarify the fact that vitamin D is not actually a vitamin, and I unravel the mysteries and myths about how our bodies take in and metabolize vitamin D.

Chapter Two: Where Does Vitamin D Come From?

In this chapter, I discuss the sources of vitamin D and review the conditions that interfere with absorbing adequate amounts from the sun. My patients have a lot of questions about getting this "sunlight vitamin" from food sources versus sunlight, tanning beds, or supplements. I answer these and I also explain why current recommended daily allowances for vitamin D are not enough to combat deficiency, much less allow us to access the optimal health benefits.

Chapter Three: Vitamin D's Role in Your Body

The purpose of this chapter is to help you make sense of the massive amount of information currently being circulated about vitamin D and its health benefits. In the last decade, the role of vitamin D has been found to have an impact on the genes, tissues, and organs of the body. Therefore, vitamin D deficiency is being linked to approximately two dozen health issues from influenza to 17 types of cancer. I also discuss the startling statistics on vitamin D deficiency in detail and highlight the impact it can have throughout the stages of your life, from infancy to maturity.

In this part of the book, I unravel the numbers associated with blood levels of vitamin D, and you will easily understand how to determine whether you are deficient or your levels are optimal. An understanding of the health implications of vitamin D deficiency is essential for making an informed decision about your own vitamin D intake.

Chapter Four: Illness, Disease, and Vitamin D Deficiency

Until recently, rickets was believed to be the only indicator of vitamin D deficiency, but current research shows that fatigue and chronic pain may also be signs. I discuss the astounding evidence that links vitamin D with cancer of the breast, colon, lung, and prostate; as well as with illnesses such as insulin-dependent diabetes, cardiovascular disease, and influenza.

Chapter Five: Measuring Vitamin D Deficiency and Optimizing Vitamin D Levels

In Chapter 5, I talk about the blood tests used to measure your levels of vitamin D, and I simplify what the numbers mean so that you can interpret your own results and empower yourself with this knowledge. You will understand more about proper dosages and why I prescribe amounts to my own patients that differ from the outdated recommendations made by the government. I talk about the safety of supplements and explain why vitamin D toxicity is extremely rare. And I also share some cautions about taking vitamin D with certain drugs or in certain circumstances.

Whom This Book Is For

I acknowledge that each of you reading this book is at a different place on your health journey. Some of you are new to vitamin supplementation, and some are seasoned supplement users. Many of you are facing health challenges and are hopeful that learning about vitamin D may help you improve your condition. My hope is that this book will reach you, no matter what your starting or launching point.

This is an important addition to your bookshelf *and* your medicine cabinet. The information in this book is essential to anyone who is interested in making positive health decisions.

This vitamin D book is for you if . . .

. . . you have been hearing about the health benefits of vitamin D and are curious about how this accessible vitamin can help you optimize your health.

. . . you want a simplified, factual version of the vitamin D story that has been in the media.

. . . your doctor or health practitioner has recommended vitamin D supplementation and you want more information.

. . . your doctor or health practitioner has warned you about the dangers of vitamin D toxicity and you want more information.

. . . you have the results from a vitamin D blood test but do not know what the numbers mean.

. . . you have some health issues and wonder if vitamin D may have health benefits for you.

. . . you are concerned about your children's health.

. . . you would like tips on how to talk to your family and loved ones about vitamin D supplementation.

. . . you would like to see the practical process I use to correct my patients' vitamin D deficiency and help them maintain their optimal levels.

If you are new to vitamin supplementation, I hope that this book will help you turn the corner from considering vitamin D supplementation to taking action.

The media reports about vitamin D have been gaining in momentum and in controversy, making a simple decision to take a vitamin fraught with debate. I have created this book as a guide to help you make safe, informed, and healthy decisions about vitamin D supplementation for you and your family.

If you have already decided to add this to your health routine, this book will validate your decision and provide you with valuable information to share with friends and loved ones. My experience with some patients has been that they leave my office eager to introduce vitamin D to their loved ones, only to be met with resistance. I offer you solid facts about supplementation as well as tips on talking to loved ones about vitamin D.

Reading this book will help you separate myth from fact. I have been talking to my patients about vitamin D for years, and in the following chapters, I have done my best to answer all of your questions about incorporating this important nutrient into your life.

Chapter One

HOW OUR UNDERSTANDING
OF VITAMIN D HAS EVOLVED

It is hard to miss the fact that vitamin D has been in the news so much lately. All of this information came out very quickly, and many of my patients were curious about the veracity of the claims being made about this vitamin. It seemed that all of a sudden, it became vitally important to overall health and mortality— it was not just about rickets and sunshine anymore. Despite the current media sound bites, the vitamin D story has been developing for centuries.

Important Discoveries Nearly 200 Years Apart

The story begins in the mid 1600s with the first mention of rickets. Rickets is a serious disease related to vitamin D deficiency. When children are vitamin D deficient, their bones do not absorb calcium and phosphorous, resulting in soft, weak, deformed bones. This same condition in adults is called osteomalacia. The first cases of rickets were documented by physicians in the 1700s as the Industrial Revolution led people from the farm to the factory. In the 19th century, the lure of factory work drew more and more people into smoggy cities, and rickets became an epidemic in Europe. It was not until 1822 that a Polish physician noted that children living in the city of Warsaw were more likely to have rickets than children living in the countryside, which led him to prescribe sunlight as a cure for the disease. This was the first link made between rickets and sunlight, but it would be another hundred years before the substance known as vitamin D was discovered.

In the 1920s and 1930s, rickets had reached epidemic proportions in North America and northern Europe. The effort was launched to find a cure, and some researchers focused their attention on food, following the lead of the Scottish Navy doctor who linked scurvy with citrus fruit in 1754. Other scientists followed up on the links made between sunlight and incidents of rickets.

Those investigating the relationship between food and rickets used cod-liver oil to cure dogs of the disease. Others investigated the relationship between sunlight, ultraviolet (UV) light, and rickets; and they found that children were cured after they were exposed to UV light. Still other researchers were investigating the chemical components of cod-liver oil, separating out the substance they believed to contain the cure. They initially theorized that vitamin A was responsible for eliminating rickets until they removed it from the cod-liver oil (leaving behind vitamin D), and it still cured the bone disease.

Despite these vital discoveries, rickets was still rampant throughout parts of the world. It was impossible to encourage people to get more sunlight when their daylight hours were spent in factories. Cod-liver oil was not catching on as the remedy that doctors were hoping for, so by the 1930s the government intervened, and bread and milk were fortified with vitamin D. Over the next 20 years, hot dogs, soda drinks, a variety of other common foods, and even beer became vitamin D fortified. Finally, food fortification led to the eradication of rickets. With the epidemic all but eliminated and no indication that vitamin D played other roles in the body, further study of the sunlight vitamin declined until the late 1960s.

The Vitamin D Toxicity Scare of the 1950s

In the 1950s, vitamin D toxicity came to the forefront in the United Kingdom when infant formulas and milk were fortified with extra, even excessive, amounts of vitamin D. This had not taken into account, however, the fact that many cereals were also fortified with extra vitamin D in a higher amount to compensate for the expected breakdown of the vitamin during storage. As a result, this led to an unfortunate epidemic of vitamin D toxicity among children.

I believe that this incident is at the root of the folklore about vitamin D being dangerous to children and harmful in large doses. Despite being reported as a vitamin D toxicity epidemic, in actuality, only several hundred children across the U.K. were affected. When the excessive fortification of food was halted, the children's symptoms disappeared. This toxicity scare led to the banning of vitamin D fortification in Europe, and this practice is linked to current cases of rickets, especially in northern parts of Europe.

I learned in medical school to be very careful when using vitamin D and was taught that since it is fat soluble, it would be easy to overdose patients. Its only real uses, my professors said, were in bone and kidney diseases. All of this information has changed, but many modern doctors and medical practitioners continue to consider vitamin D to be a potentially toxic and harmful substance, not to be taken by means other than sunlight. While I respect their caution, I also urge medical professionals to update their understanding of this essential vitamin.

◻◼◻

Doctors knew that vitamin D cured rickets but did not know how, so they began to investigate. Between 1968 and the early 1970s, researchers learned that vitamin D was metabolized in the liver and kidneys, and it controlled calcium levels in the blood through its action in the intestines. These findings led scientists to reclassify vitamin D as a hormone rather than a vitamin—a discovery that spawned yet another wave of research.

It was subsequently discovered that vitamin D receptors are found in many tissues and organs and can interact or interface with 200 or more genes that contain vitamin D response elements. Most organs in the body respond to vitamin D. This means that these cells in the organs have the ability to produce biological activities depending on the availability of vitamin D to them.

As you will learn in this book, vitamin D interacts with or affects the genes within cells throughout the body. It is being touted as a substance that may accelerate the healing of tissues and cells that may reduce the risk of cells becoming malignant.

What I know to be true is that it is not too late to reverse the vitamin D deficiency epidemic and make positive changes to your health and the health of your family.

Researchers are publishing studies and press releases, and reporters and journalists are doing their best to interpret the findings. Web-based doctors are voicing their opinions, and bloggers are posting their comments about vitamin D and its newly discovered capabilities to positively impact what some researchers call "diseases of civilization."

Since the sun-related skin-cancer scares of the 1980s, we have slathered on the sunscreen, stayed indoors, and lived with a fear of skin cancer. The fear of aging and wrinkled skin has also led to our sun avoidance. Children are spending more time inside, and when they *are* outside, they are protected from the sun with clothing and sunblock. I believe that vitamin D deficiency has risen in direct proportion to the degree in which we have avoided the sun, put on sunscreen, and moved our recreation indoors.

Researchers are discovering that illnesses and conditions ranging from autism and the common cold, to cancer and chronic pain are associated with low levels of vitamin D. I believe that I have an ethical as well as a medical and spiritual responsibility to inform as many people as possible about vitamin D and its benefits, in an effort to enhance their ability to make positive health decisions. To this end, in the next part of the book, I will provide you with significant, factual details about vitamin D.

So, What Is Vitamin D?

The first thing to understand is that it is not actually a vitamin. By definition, a vitamin is a substance that is essential to human health but cannot be produced by the body. Vitamin D, in its most obvious and fundamental function, is essential to the metabolism of calcium and phosphorous in the body. Without it, we would not have healthy bones. So it is essential to our bodies but is also produced by our bodies when we are exposed to UVB rays of the sun. Because vitamin D *is* produced by the body, it does not meet both of these criteria—therefore, it is not truly a vitamin.

Vitamin D was named a vitamin in 1920 when a researcher raised dogs without any exposure to sunlight.

He fed fish-liver oil to the animals and prevented rickets. The researcher assumed that the substance responsible for preventing the disease was in the oil—and not producible by the body. He named this essential nutrient a vitamin. It was four years later when other researchers found that vitamin D was produced in the body when exposed to sunlight. So to call vitamin D a vitamin is a misnomer, but for the benefit of public health and nutrition, as well as its name's long tradition, it is still officially *called* a vitamin.

Although the term *vitamin D* is used in reference to different substances associated with it, there are two main types of vitamin D: vitamin D_2 (known as ergocalciferol) and vitamin D_3 (also called cholecalciferol).

Which Is Better for Me . . . Vitamin D_2 or D_3?

Vitamin D_2 is produced in plants and fungi when exposed to sunlight. Ergocalciferol is not produced naturally in the human body and therefore is similar to but not identical to vitamin D_3. Most forms of ergocalciferol that we take as supplements are synthetic, and research has shown that it is significantly less effective in raising human vitamin D levels. Despite being less potent and less effective than vitamin D_3, ergocalciferol continues to be prescribed more by doctors. In fact, the only prescription vitamin D available today is vitamin D_2. Most individuals are likely to need up to twice as much vitamin D_2 as vitamin D_3.

Vitamin D_3 is naturally produced in humans and animals when sunlight hits the skin, fur, or feathers. It is the raw material from which all potent forms of vitamin D are produced in the body. Researchers agree that cholecalciferol is the more potent and effective form of vitamin D in terms of raising blood levels of vitamin D. Vitamin D_3 is generally considered safer than vitamin D_2, which has more reported cases of overdose or toxicity. There has only been one case of vitamin D_3 toxicity reported.

Important Facts about Vitamin D

Our previous understanding of the role of vitamin D was that it regulated blood levels of calcium, thus contributing to bone health. This singular role is vital, and its proper functioning keeps us alive. However, in the last ten years, researchers realized that vitamin D plays a much larger role in the maintenance of our health. In fact, it was found to have an extensive impact on the organs, tissues, and cells of the body.

Let us have a look at how vitamin D is produced in the body and the ways in which our understanding of its function has evolved over the years. I just mentioned that vitamin D is not a vitamin. So what exactly is this substance that has caught our attention so completely? In its activated form ($1,25D_3$ or calcitriol), vitamin D is a steroid hormone. It is fat soluble and can pass through cell membranes to bind to the vitamin D receptors. It is a powerful steroid hormone in the body, and it regulates gene expression by being able to affect approximately 200 genes in the body.

What It Means to Be Fat Soluble

Vitamins that are fat soluble are stored in the body for longer periods of time. Vitamin D is needed year-round, and when it is produced by UVB exposure in the summer months, it can accumulate in the body for use throughout the sunless winter. However, vitamin D can only be stored in the body if you are getting optimal amounts into your system. People who have optimal stores of vitamin D at the end of the summer can still be vitamin D deficient by the end of winter.

The Three Forms of Vitamin D

Several terms are used to refer to vitamin D in the different forms it takes on as it goes through its biochemical processes. I would like to give you a simplified version of these terms, as I will be using them throughout the rest of the book.

1. Cholecalciferol (which from now on I will call vitamin D_3) is naturally made in the body in large quantities when UVB rays hit the skin. Once you have made about 20,000 IU of vitamin D_3, a mechanism in the skin destroys excess amounts so you will not become toxic. Vitamin D_3 is available in the form of a supplement, and it is the preferred and more potent form of vitamin D, as I mentioned earlier.

2. Calcidiol (which from now on I will call 25D) is a prehormone made from the vitamin D_3 in your blood. A prehormone is a molecule that gets converted to an actual hormone. When you have your blood vitamin D levels measured, you must have the 25D levels tested. Another term that the labs will use for this form of vitamin D is 25-hydroxyvitamin D. Be aware of which vitamin D test your doctor is ordering for you.

3. Calcitriol (which from now on I will call $1,25D_3$) is also made from vitamin D_3 and is a potent steroid hormone manufactured in many cells, tissues, and organs in the body. This is the active form of vitamin D that researchers are excited about because of its many additional properties. Some doctors may mistakenly order a vitamin D blood test measuring $1,25D_3$, but this will not accurately assess your level of vitamin D deficiency. The $1,25D_3$ in the blood comes from the kidneys and does not reflect how much vitamin D is in other organs.

How Do We Get Our Vitamin D?

Step 1: The sun hits your skin or you take a vitamin D_3 supplement. If you are using the sun as your source of vitamin D, the process begins when the skin is exposed to the sun. The UVB light in the sun interfaces with a form of cholesterol in your skin called 7-dehydrocholesterol, and this substance is synthesized into pre–vitamin D_3. The pre–vitamin D_3 immediately converts into vitamin D_3. This is the vitamin D that circulates through the body, but it still is not empowered into its activated form.

Vitamin D_3 is made in large quantities when you are in the sun during peak UV times. In fact, it is estimated

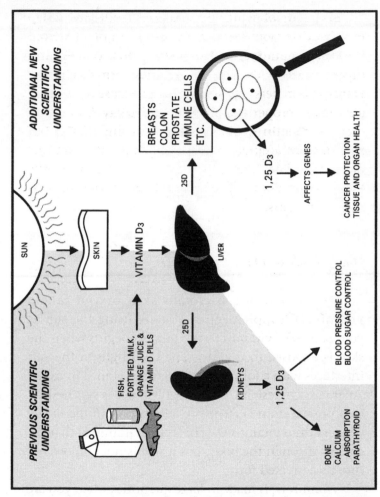

Figure 1. Previous and Newly Recognized Understanding of Vitamin D Actions

that in the summertime, if you spend 30 minutes in the midday sun in a bathing suit, you can make up to 20,000 IU of vitamin D. Remember, if you get too much sun, the skin is able to convert the excess vitamin D to other inactive molecules. Because of this, the body does not get overdosed with vitamin D from sun exposure.

For my patients who do not get enough sun, I advise them to take vitamin D as a supplement in carefully selected dosages.

Step 2: Vitamin D_3 becomes 25D (see Figure 1). From your sun exposure or supplements, the vitamin D_3 makes its way to the liver where it undergoes a process (hydroxylation), turning it into 25D to store in your body. Having optimal stores of 25D in your body is very important, as these stores will enhance your body's ability to make the best use of vitamin D's capabilities. If your body does not store enough vitamin D in the form of 25D, then you will have low or deficient levels in the blood. Ideally, your vitamin D level should be optimal.

Step 3: 25D becomes $1,25D_3$. The first priority for the health of your body is to send 25D from your liver to the kidneys, where it is transformed into $1,25D_3$, which is the active and potent form of vitamin D. Its job is to circulate in your blood to ensure that you maintain appropriate levels of calcium. This function of $1,25D_3$ is vital to your health—so much so that scientists did not expect it to have other functions.

In 1998, vitamin D researcher Michael Holick, M.D., Ph.D., and his colleagues discovered that the kidneys were not the only place in the body where 25D was metabolized into the potent and vital substance $1,25D_3$. When your body has enough stores of 25D and has maintained the proper functioning of calcium levels in the blood, something exciting happens to the "excess" 25D.

It is only in the last ten years that scientists have come to understand this newfound function of the 25D form of vitamin D. They have discovered that most tissues and cells of the body have the ability to metabolize 25D from the liver and turn it into $1,25D_3$. When researchers discovered these extra steps in the metabolizing of vitamin D, they realized that many organs, tissues, and cells in the body have receptors for vitamin D. This means that vitamin D circulates throughout the body and has the ability to land and affect the cells, tissues, and organs that receive the vitamin D. It is the only substance of its kind in the body, and researchers are finding that it has many repair and maintenance functions in most tissues and cells. Vitamin D is not just about healthy bones anymore.

It is this new fact about the $1,25D_3$ form of vitamin D that has researchers so excited. According to John Cannell, M.D., $1,25D_3$ affects more than 200 genes and can be found in most tissues in the body. He states on his Website: "This explains why the same substance may have a role in preventing cancer, influenza, autism, asthma, multiple sclerosis, and cardiovascular disease, not just curing rickets, and osteomalacia."

In his recent book *The UV Advantage,* vitamin D researcher Dr. Michael Holick said, "Can you imagine what would happen if one of the drug companies came out with a single pill that reduced the risk of cancer, heart attack, stroke, osteoporosis, PMS, seasonal affective disorder, and various autoimmune disorders? There would be a media frenzy the likes of which has never been seen in response to a medical breakthrough!"

I could not agree more and I am happy to tell you that such a pill exists! It is called vitamin D, and it is everywhere—it is available to you right now without a prescription and for just pennies a tablet.

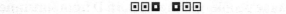

Chapter Two

WHERE DOES VITAMIN D COME FROM?

We get our vitamin D from several sources: the sun, as I have just discussed; the foods we eat; and the supplements we take. Tanning beds are another way to get vitamin D. My goal here is to provide an overview of the current status of vitamin D sources.

Vitamin D from the Sun

For some people, getting vitamin D from sunshine alone feels like the right and natural choice. For others, sun exposure is a scary thing and is avoided at all costs; these individuals spend more time indoors and wear protective clothing or sunscreen when outside. And some, especially those who live in sunny climates, assume that they are getting adequate levels of vitamin D when they step outside for a few minutes.

Let me provide you with more information about getting vitamin D from the sun, as there are facts to consider that you might not have thought about before. It may not be as easy as you think to get enough vitamin D into your system to achieve optimal health benefits.

Two kinds of ultraviolet (UV) light pass through the ozone layer on their way to earth—and your skin. It is important to know the difference between the two types of rays: UVA and UVB.

— **UVA rays** are long rays from the sun. They do not cause sunburn, but they penetrate more deeply into your skin and contribute to premature aging, discoloration, and wrinkles. UVA rays are active at all times of the day and throughout the year. They pass through glass and clothing but do not prompt your skin to produce vitamin D.

— **UVB rays** are important in two ways. First, the UVB rays are responsible for turning your skin red and causing sunburn. Second, when UVB rays hit your skin, they launch the production of vitamin D. Do you see the conflict here? This is the biological mechanism at the root of the sunshine debate that has been spawned by discussions of vitamin D deficiency. The question remains: how do we recommend getting vitamin D?

Plus, there is a very limited wavelength of solar UVB light (290–315 nanometers) that actually causes the creation of vitamin D in the body. If the UVB rays are outside that limited frequency, vitamin D will not be made by the body.

Vitamin D Tip

UVB rays cannot penetrate glass or clothing, so you do not produce vitamin D just by sitting near a window.

The Sunshine Conundrum

We live in a time where sun exposure is considered by some to be a health menace. In an effort to prevent skin cancer, dermatologists have done an amazing job of encouraging people of all ages to don sunscreen and protective clothing and spend more time in shaded areas. Children are covered in sunscreen from their first foray into the sunshine.

However, in this effort to protect us from the possibility of skin cancer, we have cut ourselves off from a vital source of health—vitamin D. Why would anyone take a step into the sun when we have been warned for 20 years that it is a health hazard?

In addition to the fear of skin cancer, anti-aging proponents are warning us about sun damage to the skin in the form of wrinkles. So we have been driven from the sun for the sake of health and vanity. It is so confusing for many who are reading and hearing about the health benefits of vitamin D. Many want to make some positive health choices, but they are stuck in the doorway—even hesitating to venture forth into the sun to buy some vitamin D supplements!

Defining the International Unit (IU)

The international unit (IU) is a unit of measurement based on an accepted standard and on biological activity of the substance. The IU for vitamin D is unique to this substance—that is, 100 IU of vitamin D does not equal 100 IU of vitamin E. 1,000 IU of vitamin D equals 25 micrograms (mcg) of vitamin D.

The fact remains that the sun *is* a great way to get vitamin D—it is "the sunshine vitamin," after all. It is even the preferred way to absorb phenomenal amounts into your system quickly. Just 12 minutes of summer noonday sun with bare arms and legs would provide a white woman on average with approximately 3,000 IU of vitamin D; and in less than 30 minutes, she could have up to 20,000 IU! However, many of my patients have told me that exposure to the sun just is not practical for them, as they are very conscious of avoiding a sunburn and sun damage, in addition to their concerns about skin cancer.

I want to help you understand how, when, and under what circumstances the sun is able to create vitamin D in the skin. With this information, I hope that you will be able to make informed decisions on how to best get your vitamin D.

Conditions That Interfere with Getting Enough Vitamin D from the Sun

There are so many factors influencing the degree in which you can get adequate amounts of vitamin D from sun exposure that I recommend that my patients be on the safe side . . . and take vitamin D supplements in conjunction with monitoring their blood levels through testing. I will discuss those details later, but right now, I want to explain why the sun is a complicated topic.

The following is a list of factors that come between you and vitamin D–producing UVB rays. The first six are about your environment, and the last five concern you. The important thing to keep in mind as you are reading is that each of these conditions inherently contributes to an increased risk of having a vitamin D deficiency and thereby increases your chances of developing an illness or disease that is associated with vitamin D deficiency (these are discussed in Chapter 4).

1. Latitude
2. Season of the year
3. Altitude
4. Time of day
5. Air pollution
6. Cloud cover
7. Use of sunblock
8. Melanin content of the skin
9. Age
10. Weight
11. Amount of clothing covering the body

1. Latitude

Any discussion about vitamin D and vitamin D deficiency involves having an understanding of the impact of latitude on sun exposure—on vitamin D—and ultimately its effect on certain illnesses and diseases. Latitude is measured in degrees north and south, representing the distance between a specific place and the equator. The equator is at zero degrees latitude, and the sun is directly overhead; therefore, the sun's UV rays have the shortest distance to travel to reach the earth's surface. New York City is at 40 degrees latitude; and Flagstaff, Arizona, is at 35 degrees latitude. In both of these cities, the sun is significantly lower in the sky than it is in places located closer to the equator.

When the sun is lower in the sky (at higher latitudes), the UV rays have a longer distance to travel to reach the earth's surface. In addition, the sun's rays must make their way through thicker ozone and cloud cover in order to reach your skin. When the sun is higher in the sky (at lower latitudes), the UV rays have a shorter distance and a clearer path to the earth's surface.

As a reference point, the North Pole is 90 degrees north latitude with the sun very low in the sky. The higher your latitude, the less intense the UV rays and the lower your access to the UVB rays that prompt your skin to make vitamin D.

Determining Your Latitude

To determine your latitude, you can use a GPS (global positioning system). Google Earth has a built-in function that displays the latitude for spots on the map that you point to with your cursor.

Here is the important point to remember: If you live above 35 degrees latitude, you will not be able to make vitamin D from the sun from approximately November to March, no matter how long you are exposed. Unfortunately, there is no way around this fact. When you look at a map of North America, fully two-thirds of the United States and all of Canada is above 35 degrees latitude.

Cities Near the 35 Degrees Latitude Mark
Albuquerque, NM
Amarillo, TX
Bakersfield, CA
Charlotte, NC
Flagstaff, AZ
Knoxville, TN
Memphis, TN
Oklahoma City, OK
Raleigh, NC
Santa Fe, NM

As a reference point for my Canadian readers, part of the border between the United States and Canada is nicknamed the 49th parallel. Every city between Vancouver, B.C., and Winnipeg, Manitoba, is above 49 degrees latitude. East of Manitoba, the lowest latitudes are 43 degrees in southern Ontario and the southern tip of Nova Scotia.

The fact that the incidence of many illnesses and diseases escalates with the increase in latitude has catapulted the research on sun exposure, vitamin D deficiency, and illness. As you will learn later in this book, much of the research on vitamin D and illness has launched from the understanding of the implications of latitude.

Even if you are living in a lower latitude and can make vitamin D throughout the year, there are still several other factors that interfere with vitamin D production, as you will see as you read about the following factors.

2. Season of the Year

The season of the year affects the angle at which the sun hits the earth, and that angle affects how much UVB gets through to your skin. Without UVB rays on your skin, you cannot make vitamin D. So the amount of vitamin D you can produce from the sun will fluctuate with the seasons. Generally speaking, most people with average exposure to the sun will have higher vitamin D levels at the end of summer than at the end of winter.

Your particular vitamin D season will change according to your latitude. If you live in Boston, which is at 42 degrees latitude, you may have access to UVB rays (depending on the other factors discussed) from April to October. But in the winter—from November to March—if you are living above 35 degrees latitude, you will not get *any* vitamin D from the sun in these months. No matter how long you sit in the sun in the middle of winter above 35 degrees latitude, your skin will not produce any vitamin D.

Summer Sunshine Does Not Guarantee Sufficient Vitamin D!

A study conducted in Boston revealed that 36 percent of the young men and women who participated in the study were deficient in vitamin D at the *end* of the summer. Among those who were over age 50, 42 percent were vitamin D deficient—at the end of summer!

As you go farther north, the number of vitamin D–producing days per year decreases. If you are gathering sufficient sun in the summer to elevate your vitamin D levels and store it in your fat, the question remains whether or not that will be enough to keep your levels optimal throughout the winter. If you live somewhere with long winters, you are likely to experience low vitamin D levels at the same time each year. Some have called this phenomenon the "vitamin D winter." In some areas in Norway that sit at 70 degrees latitude, part of their long UVB-free winter coincides with cod season, and residents are able to replenish their vitamin D stores by eating cod livers.

3. Altitude

At lower altitudes, the ultraviolet radiation from the sun is absorbed by the atmosphere and is therefore less intense than at higher altitudes. People living at low altitudes will have less access to the UVB rays that help them make vitamin D. Those who live in the mountains will have greater access to the UVB rays needed to make vitamin D.

4. Time of Day

Weather reports often detail the UV Index—a number rating the ultraviolet radiation from the sun at specific hours of the day. The higher the rating, the more likely you are to burn in the sun. Researchers have found that your ability to make vitamin D from the sun increases with the UV Index. In some seasons and latitudes, the only time you will be able to produce vitamin D would be between 10 A.M. and 2 P.M. or when the UV Index is at least a 3. While it might be sunny for the rest of the day, these are the hours when vitamin D–making UVB rays are most potent. You can find information about the UV Index in your area from searching the Internet for your current weather.

5. Air Pollution

Pollution in the air can block UVB rays from the sun, thereby inhibiting your ability to make vitamin D. In one study in India, blood levels of people living in areas with high air pollution had 54 percent less vitamin D than those residing in areas with little air pollution. Of the children tested in the polluted areas, 46 percent had deficient levels of vitamin D, and 12 percent of the children had rickets.

6. Cloud Cover

UVB light, which is necessary for the production of vitamin D, is cut in half by cloud cover.

7. Use of Sunblock

Sunblock and sunscreen prevent UVB rays (and sometimes UVA rays) from being absorbed by the skin. The higher the SPF (Sun Protection Factor), the more protected you are from the sun's harmful rays as well as the vitamin D–producing rays. A sunscreen with an SPF 8 prevents up to 92 percent of your skin's production of vitamin D, whereas sunscreen with an SPF 15 cuts it by up to 99 percent. The heightening debate is whether protecting your skin from the harmful rays of the sun is also putting you at a higher risk for developing illnesses associated with vitamin D deficiency.

I suggest to my patients that they spend a few minutes in the sun before applying sunblock. This way the skin can produce some vitamin D before being shielded from UV rays. I will talk more about this later in the book.

8. Melanin Content of the Skin

The fact that surprises my patients most is that the darker your skin, the less vitamin D your body produces from sun exposure. In fact, people with dark or black skin are at greater risk for being deficient because it is harder for them to produce vitamin D in the skin. And for those who get suntans, their tanned skin also blocks the UVB rays from creating vitamin D.

Melanin is the pigment in your skin that gives you color, and it absorbs the UVB rays, inhibiting vitamin D production. People with dark or black skin need intense sunlight to penetrate the skin in order to make vitamin D—up to 10 times the amount of sun that light-skinned people require. This worked well during the times when the melanin content of people's skin matched the latitudes they lived in. For example, when people with dark skin lived close to the equator, they were able to gather the necessary rays to produce vitamin D. People with paler skin lived in northern latitudes where there was less sun and more cloud cover. But because individuals with light skin can make vitamin D with less sun exposure, they got sufficient amounts of UVB.

In 1975, Thomas Fitzpatrick, a Harvard medical doctor, developed a system to classify people's skin type based on their complexion and the skin's response to sun exposure. There are six skin types according to this classification.

What Is Your Skin Type?	
Type 1	Skin always burns, never tans, and is extremely fair.
Type 2	Skin always burns, occasionally tans, and is considered fair.
Type 3	Skin occasionally burns, gradually tans, and is considered medium.
Type 4	Skin rarely burns, always tans, and is considered olive.
Type 5	Skin seldom burns, always tans, and is considered medium to dark.
Type 6	Skin never burns, always tans darkly, and is considered dark.

Many studies have shown that African-American people have staggering rates of vitamin D deficiency. Not only is the incidence of deficiency high (with some studies indicating that all participants—100 percent—were vitamin D deficient), but their degree of deficiency is extremely high.

Ironically, people who are normally light skinned but spend time tanning may actually produce more melanin in their skin, thus reducing their ability to convert the sunlight into vitamin D.

9. Age

Elderly people are also at higher risk for developing vitamin D deficiency. As we age, we produce less of the vitamin D precursor in our skin and therefore produce less vitamin D when we are exposed to the sun. Studies also show that elderly individuals spend less time in the sun, whether from fear of skin cancer or because their outdoor activity is inhibited. Lack of sun exposure disables their vitamin D production.

Older People Need More Sun Exposure to Make Vitamin D

If an elderly person is in the sun for the same length of time as a young person, the older individual will produce merely 25 percent of the vitamin D that the younger person is able to produce.

10. Weight

People who are overweight have trouble making enough vitamin D from the sun. Vitamin D is a fat-soluble vitamin, so fat cells absorb it, making it less available for use in tissues and organs throughout the body. One study indicated that obese people had blood levels of vitamin D that were 57 percent lower than lean subjects exposed to the same levels of vitamin D–making UVB.

11. Amount of Clothing Covering the Body

Evolution-wise, humans started out not wearing many clothes. As we evolved into clothes-wearing beings, our access to appropriate levels of sunshine decreased with the number of articles of clothing that we donned. Clothing is obviously effective as a protection from the rays of the sun. Dermatologists and cancer specialists recommend wearing sunglasses, hats, and long-sleeved shirts to offer the most protection. In addition, cultural apparel, which includes clothing that fully covers the body, definitely creates a barrier between the skin and the sun. For example, women and children in Saudi Arabia have high rates of rickets, osteomalacia, and vitamin D deficiency. Because their bodies are completely concealed, their skin does not come into contact with UVB rays. People living in similar sunny regions who do not wear cultural apparel, and are therefore able to manufacture vitamin D from the sun's UVB rays, will have significantly higher levels of vitamin D.

How Much Sun Would I Need to Increase My Vitamin D Level?

The amount of sun exposure you need to elevate the level of vitamin D in your system differs drastically from person to person. That is the short answer to the question. I mentioned earlier that a woman with white skin and bare arms and legs only needed 12 minutes of summer midday sun to load up on approximately 3,000 IU of vitamin D. On the other end of the spectrum, a similarly dressed woman with black skin may need up to 10 times the sun exposure to get the same amount of vitamin D—that is spending up to two hours in the sun to get only 3,000 IU of vitamin D. Sun exposure is complicated!

Vitamin D researcher Michael Holick, M.D., Ph.D., has described a way to obtain between 800 and 1,500 IU of vitamin D from the sun. He refers to the term minimal erythemal dose (MED), which describes how much time it takes for *your* skin to turn pink in the sun. Dr. Holick's formula for safe exposure to the sun is to expose 25 percent of your skin (hands, arms, and lower legs) to the sun for 25 to 50 percent of the time you would estimate it would take for your skin to turn pink from the sun (MED). For example, if you are fair skinned, your skin may turn pink within ten minutes of being in the sun. If you stayed in the sun without wearing sunblock for 25 to 50 percent of your MED (2.5 to 5 minutes), you would gather about 1,000 IU of vitamin D. Dr. Holick recommends doing this a few times a week during the times of year when you can get access to UVB rays. But if you have turned pink—you have had too much sun!

The 11 factors I have just described highlight the complications of maneuvering in and out of the sun in an effort to get adequate vitamin D safely from sun alone. Having even one of these factors in your reality will increase your risk of vitamin D deficiency. So instead of teaching my patients to choreograph their latitude and season, time of day, melanin, MED, and clothing in order to get their optimal amounts of vitamin D, I teach them about proper testing and supplementation.

Obtaining Vitamin D from Food

Some health experts and nutritionists insist that we can get sufficient amounts of vitamin D by eating foods that are rich in this substance. There is much conflicting data about the presence of vitamin D in food. Some avid proponents of healthy eating cling to the belief that all of our nutrition can come from eating a balanced and healthy diet. While this ideal is admirable, there are a few considerations about diet that remain a fact for most people.

You Cannot Eat Enough Fish, Eggs, or Mushrooms to Get Adequate—Let Alone Optimal—Amounts of Vitamin D

- If "food experts" do not know that the vitamin D content in food is inadequate to reap health benefits, how can the average person be expected to know about the vitamin D content in food?

- Most people do not eat healthy, balanced diets and will never achieve adequate vitamin D levels from diet alone.

- There simply are not enough foods that naturally contain amounts of vitamin D that will raise your blood level to an optimal rate.

- Foods fortified with vitamin D do not contain uniform amounts of the substance and may not contain the amount of vitamin D reported on the packaging.

Facts about Fortified Food

In many American and Canadian households during the winter, the vitamin D in fortified food provides up to 85 percent of total vitamin D intake. For decades, fortified food has made vitamin D accessible to people of all ages throughout North America. However, the current amount contained in fortified food will never be enough to combat the levels of deficiency we are currently experiencing.

Food is fortified with vitamin D_2 or the preferred vitamin D_3, which is more potent than D_2. Milk, orange juice, margarine, some cereals, and products made from fortified milk are the basic foods that are fortified with vitamin D. In Canada, only margarine and milk are mandated to be fortified with vitamin D. For those who are lactose intolerant or who avoid drinking milk, there are not many alternatives.

Although fortified, these foods and drinks contain very small quantities of vitamin D. Therefore, you have to consume large quantities of the food regularly to get enough vitamin D. For example, in order to obtain a mere 1,000 IU in a day, you would have to drink ten eight-ounce glasses of milk. Many families rely on milk to get their vitamin D, but I can guarantee that they are not getting enough from milk alone.

The accuracy of the vitamin D measured in milk has also been called into question. One study verified that most of the milk sampled contained less than 20 percent of the listed amount. Batches of milk of the same brand varied in vitamin D content on different days.

Cod-liver oil is commonly recommended as a source of vitamin D. It is true that it contains vitamin D, but it also has a large amount of vitamin A. In order to use cod-liver oil to take in the amount of vitamin D that I recommend, you would end up getting an overdose of vitamin A, which can be toxic.

While reading about vitamin D in the media and popular press in the preparation of this book, I was surprised by the number of blogs, news reports, and Website commentaries that focus on the topic of food as a source of vitamin D. I was even more surprised to read the recommendations by credentialed nutritionists advocating that people rely exclusively on food for their vitamin D supply.

The following table from the National Institutes of Health, Office of Dietary Supplements Website lists the foods that contain vitamin D. Please note that these foods include those with naturally occurring vitamin D and those fortified with vitamin D.

National Institutes of Health, Office of Dietary Supplements	
Food	Vit. D IUs per serving
Cod-liver oil, 1 tablespoon	1,360
Salmon, cooked, 3.5 ounces	360
Mackerel, cooked, 3.5 ounces	345
Tuna fish, canned in oil, 3 ounces	200
Sardines, canned in oil, drained, 1.75 ounces	250
Milk, nonfat, reduced fat, and whole, vitamin D–fortified, 1 cup	98
Margarine, fortified, 1 tablespoon	60
Ready-to-eat cereal, fortified with 10 percent of the daily RDA for vitamin D, 0.75–1 cup	40
Egg, 1 whole (vitamin D is found in yolk)	20
Liver, beef, cooked, 3.5 ounces	15
Cheese, Swiss, 1 ounce	12

The Recommended Daily Allowance (or Recommended Dietary Allowance) (RDA) is the amount of a nutrient that is deemed necessary by the government to maintain health. The recommendations are made by the Food and Nutrition Board of the National Research Council of The National Academy of Sciences in the U.S., and the amounts recommended are intended to meet the requirements of 98 percent of the healthy population.

2008 RDA in the United States

Currently in the United States, the RDA for vitamin D for people up to age 49 is 200 IU per day, and 400 IU per day for those over 50. The upper-limit safe dose of vitamin D was set at 2,000 IU per day. The majority of vitamin D researchers feel that these levels are woefully inadequate.

The current (2008) RDA levels for vitamin D were developed in 1997 and set at a level to prevent rickets and other bone diseases. They were not set to prevent vitamin D deficiency as we understand it now. There has been an abundance of research studies since 1997 that consistently report a decreased incidence of illness and disease with higher blood levels of vitamin D. In response to these scientific findings, many nutrition and health experts including myself are calling for an increase in the RDA levels for vitamin D so that these higher levels can be maintained.

Studies published in 2001 verified that the current recommended daily allowance of vitamin D will not prevent vitamin D deficiency as defined in today's medical literature. So even if you are diligent about taking your multivitamin containing 400 IU of vitamin D or eating vitamin D–rich foods, you will not prevent vitamin D deficiency. You may not contract rickets or osteomalacia—but quite likely, you will still have deficient levels of vitamin D.

In my opinion and in the opinion of many of my colleagues, the government's RDA is not enough to combat deficiency. Because it was set in 1997, the current RDA does not take into account the accumulating research that shows the health benefits of optimal blood levels of vitamin D. Many sources indicate that experts are calling for government action to increase the RDA.

How Is the Upper Limit of the RDA Decided?

In a recent interview, Dr. Cedric Garland talked about how the government derived the maximum level, or upper limit of safety of vitamin D. He explained that when the government representatives meet to set the recommended maximum levels of a substance like vitamin D, their job is to set the limit to eliminate the possibility of any negative health effects. The organization is very invested in reducing the risk of toxicity. The recommended maximum levels are different from the RDA—this number represents the most vitamin D that anyone should take in a day. According to Garland, the team of experts set 4,800 IU as the lowest dose in which there was any perceivable negative health effect. In the interest of safety, that number was cut in half. So the maximum upper limit—to be safe—is actually down to 2,400 IU/day. To be even safer, they took off another 400 IU/day. This is how the upper limit of 2,000 IU/day was decided, and that was based on the research available more than ten years ago, when the recommendations for vitamin D were only for the maintenance of healthy, strong bones.

The conservative upper limits recommended by the government did not make sense to me when I realized that 30 minutes of sun exposure in the middle of the day can increase our vitamin D by as much as 20,000 IU—so if Mother Nature has chosen to give us such a large dose from sun exposure, how could 4,800 be harmful?

In order to get your 2,000 IU per day of vitamin D from food, you would have to consume 5.5 servings— nearly 20 ounces of salmon every day or 20 cups of fortified milk. Or you would have to spend time with a calculator and the Internet to figure out how to safely get 2,000 IU of vitamin D from the sun.

Other Sources of UVB Rays

Tanning Beds as a Source of UVB Rays

The machines used in tanning facilities emit radiation in the form of UVB and UVA rays. The UVB rays are responsible for the skin's manufacturing of vitamin D. These rays are also responsible for sunburn, risk of skin cancer, and premature aging. While the machines are a viable source of UVB rays, their use is so controversial that I am not prepared to make a recommendation about using them. UVA rays do not cause sunburn but penetrate the skin deeply, contributing to premature aging of the skin and wrinkles, as well as skin cancer.

Dr. Michael Holick has extensively researched the safety of sun and UVB exposure, which includes the use of tanning beds. I recommend consulting his book for his specific guidelines. He insists that you pay the same attention to timing your tanning-bed use as you do to your sun exposure. As I have mentioned, Dr. Holick recommends attaining 25 to 50 percent of MED (the length of time it would take your skin to turn pink) several times a week as the maximum amount of exposure.

The whole area of exposure to UVB rays and the sun is controversial, but I do believe that safe sun exposure is a good way to get vitamin D. However, because most dermatologists and their national societies are so against it, it is not the primary way I recommend that my patients obtain their vitamin D.

Supplements as a Form of Vitamin D

While sunshine is still the richest source of vitamin D, as I just noted, it is often impractical to get adequate sun exposure. Supplements, which come in the form of vitamin D_2 and D_3, are my preferred source. Some experts are concerned that if the public is told that a little vitamin D supplementation is good, then the consumer will think that more is even better. Until recently, there were very few sources for vitamin D in doses more than 400 IU. Many people were getting their 400 IU/day by taking a multivitamin containing that amount (which is the RDA). The concern was that people were attempting to increase their daily intake of vitamin D by taking more multivitamins, thereby exposing themselves to toxic levels of other vitamins, especially vitamin A.

If you are taking medications and antibiotics that cause sun sensitivity, your physician may have recommended complete sun avoidance. Vitamin D supplementation is something that I recommend to my patients who are avoiding the sun, and I will describe my supplementation process in greater detail later in the book.

Chapter Three

VITAMIN D'S ROLE IN YOUR BODY

In this chapter, I am going to talk about vitamin D deficiency and its implications for your own health and that of your family. In the last decade, enthusiastic scientists have found that vitamin D has an impact on the genes, tissues, and organs of the body. This is an important, even vital, finding.

In our history with vitamin D, we have assumed that its only role was to prevent rickets in children and help them form healthy bones. Essentially, if someone did not have a bone disease such as rickets, osteomalacia, or osteoporosis, vitamin D deficiency was not given any consideration. Once we passed childhood, we did not think about vitamin D deficiency again.

Vitamin D Is Found in Most Tissues in the Body

Earlier in the book, I told you how vitamin D was processed in the liver and then circulated in the body as 25D.

The first priority for the body is for the kidneys to grab the 25D and turn it into $1,25D_3$, which is the vital, active form of vitamin D. This $1,25D_3$ circulates in the blood and interacts with intestinal cells to stimulate the absorption of calcium. This maintains your blood calcium levels, which in turn keeps your bones hard and strong. This is the fundamental function of vitamin D because you need it to help you absorb calcium. Until recently, this was believed to be the *only* job of vitamin D. We now know that the average person requires vitamin D blood levels of at least 30 ng/ml in order to optimize the ability of the body to absorb calcium in the intestines.

In the early 1990s it was found that the activated vitamin D had anti-cancer properties. At that time it was believed that the kidneys processed all of the 25D and that they were the only organs able to convert it to the activated $1,25D$ D_3, which then got transported throughout the body. The theory was that the more vitamin D you had in your body, the more the kidneys would process and make available in this activated form for the benefit of the rest of the body.

It is only in the last decade that scientists have proven that most all of the organs in the body also have the ability to process the 25D from the liver into its active form, vitamin $1,25D_3$. (See Figure 1, Chapter 1.) It is as if there are landing pads, called vitamin D receptors (VDR) in most of the organs of the body. If there is extra vitamin D (25D) in your body after the kidneys do their job maintaining calcium, then that 25D will be transported throughout the body to be converted to $1,25D_3$, within each organ.

In this activated form, vitamin D has unique functions depending on the needs of the cells and tissues it is in. The amazing thing is that the $1,25D_3$ that is created in these other organs does not enter the body's circulation; rather, it is utilized by the cells of that organ and then immediately broken down within the organ. That is why it took so long for researchers to discover this new $1,25D_3$ because it was hiding inside the organs. This mechanism also prevents the body from letting too much $1,25D_3$ into the bloodstream where it could affect calcium metabolism.

Among other things, $1,25D_3$ has been found to contain powerful properties linked to cancer prevention. If you do not have enough 25D stored in your body, then you will not be able to get the benefit of this important mechanism of organ $1,25D_3$ production.

If the average person needs vitamin D blood levels of at least 30 ng/ml to carry out the fundamental job of calcium absorption, an individual will require higher levels of vitamin D to get these new health benefits.

Vitamin D Levels—What the Numbers Mean

The only way to determine your level of vitamin D is to get a blood test to measure the amount of 25D in your blood. This is the form of vitamin D that is processed in the liver—not the activated form of vitamin D $(1,25D_3)$. The typical normal range in standard vitamin D blood tests is just over 20 ng/ml. As you will learn later, researchers now believe that you need a vitamin D blood level of at least 30 to 40 ng/ml in order to activate these newly discovered functions.

In my practice, in order to determine the relative vitamin D status of my patients, I follow guidelines identified by integrative-medicine practitioners as outlined in the following chart.

Levels of Vitamin D
Less than 10 ng/ml: Severe deficiency
10–20 ng/ml: Deficiency
20–30 ng/ml: Insufficiency
30 ng/ml and above: "Normal"
40–70 ng/ml: Optimal (at the time of this writing)
Over 100 ng/ml: Overdose
Over 150 ng/ml: Toxic

I am striving to help all of my patients optimize their vitamin D levels; in other words, I work with them to elevate their vitamin D to be between 40 and 70 ng/ml.

Math Tip

Note that the current unit of measurement for vitamin D levels in the blood is expressed in ng/ml: nanograms per milliliter. You may see other authors using another measurement expressed in nmol/l, which is nanomoles per liter. To change ng/ml to nmol/l, multiply by 2.5. For example, 40 ng/ml equals 100 nmol/l.

The Startling Statistics of Vitamin D Deficiency

In 2004, it was estimated that the economic burden of vitamin D deficiency due to inadequate access to the sun, supplements, diet, and food fortification cost the U.S. from $40 to $56 billion annually. In 2007, researchers Grant, Garland, and Gorham estimated that it would cost $1 billion each year to provide all adult Americans with 1,000 IU of vitamin D daily. They also estimated that in the United States, the daily provision of 1,000 IU of vitamin D would reduce cancer mortality for females by 9 percent and 7 percent for males. The researchers estimated that this would reduce the country's annual cost of cancer treatment by $16 to $25 billion.

The researchers also made estimates for Western European countries below 59 degrees latitude: Cancer mortality rates could reduce by 20 percent for females and 14 percent for men.

Worldwide, it is estimated that one billion people have deficient or insufficient levels of vitamin D. References from a number of studies indicate that in North America and northern Europe, between 40 and 100 percent of elderly people are deficient in vitamin D. The *Mayo Clinic Proceedings* reported on a study from Minnesota that 100 percent of African Americans, East Africans, Hispanics, and American Indians in the study were vitamin D deficient. In addition, more than 50 percent of postmenopausal women who have osteoporosis bad enough that they required prescription medication had insufficient levels of 25D (below 30 ng/ml). One can only guess how much this impacts the amount of money spent on medical treatments. This is one of the reasons why I believe it is my responsibility to help my patients reach optimal vitamin D levels.

Sun Avoidance and Vitamin D Deficiency

Since the late 1980s, we have been told to stay out of the sun to reduce the risk of skin cancer and avoid premature skin aging. Medical groups such as dermatologists advised people to avoid sun exposure and always wear sunscreen when they do spend time outdoors. However, these sweeping warnings about the sun's dangers were not accompanied by the recommendation to increase vitamin D supplementation. We were avoiding the sun in droves but not replenishing our vitamin D. Not only have we become deficient, but vitamin D experts are beginning to link this deficiency with the rise of the illnesses of modern society.

In evolutionary terms, humans have evolved from living naked near the equator and migrating to the northern hemispheres to where we cover ourselves with clothing year-round. In comparison to our distant ancestors, we are sun starved and therefore vitamin D starved. Our ancestors, bathed in sun for much of the day, probably had naturally occurring levels of vitamin D in their blood between 50 and 90 ng/ml. In my busy medical practice, in five years of testing 25D levels, I have only seen a few people with optimal levels of vitamin D on initial testing.

In my experience, counting on patients to get enough sunshine on a regular basis is not enough to help them elevate their vitamin D levels to optimal rates. This is why I recommend supplementation, and I will talk about specific dosages that I have prescribed for my patients in Chapter 5.

What Is Your Risk for Vitamin D Deficiency?

At this point, you are probably wondering about your chances of being vitamin D deficient. The short answer is that it is very likely that you do not have sufficient stores of vitamin D in your system to achieve the optimal health benefits associated with it. In my medical practice, I have estimated that over 75 percent of my new patients are deficient or insufficient in vitamin D.

In Chapter 2, I described the factors that interfere with you getting adequate exposure to the appropriate amount and type of sun. Naturally, those conditions also heighten the risk of vitamin D deficiency. In addition to low sun exposure due to latitude, weather, season, skin color, and concealing clothing, there are other factors that can increase your risk of vitamin D deficiency.

Part of the greatest risk for vitamin D deficiency is that no one expects to have a vitamin D deficiency! If people made it through childhood without contracting rickets, it is believed that they are in the clear. If you do not have rickets or osteomalacia, how do you know if you are deficient? Vitamin D deficiency has been termed a silent epidemic because the symptoms associated with vitamin D deficiency are more subtle and can be confused with many other medical conditions. Many doctors do not test for it unless bone problems are suspected. I test all of my new patients for it as part of their initial workup.

Interestingly, more studies are linking the symptoms associated with many diseases of civilization with vitamin D deficiency. If you have any of the following common complaints, you may be vitamin D deficient:

- Muscular weakness
- Feeling of heaviness in the legs
- Chronic musculoskeletal pain
- Fatigue or easy tiring
- Frequent infections
- Depression

A Case of Neck Pain and Low Vitamin D Levels

In my practice, many patients with similar complaints have reported a decrease in their symptoms after following my supplementation protocol. In one such example, I saw a middle-aged physician who experienced persistent neck pain for some years. He had received regular chiropractic adjustments, body work, and acupuncture; and would use occasional ibuprofen for his neck pain.

He came to me approximately five years ago when I was first measuring vitamin D levels. His vitamin D blood level was at 11 ng/ml! This was significantly deficient, and I immediately started him on a corrective dose of vitamin D to bring his level up quickly.

After taking vitamin D for approximately six weeks, the patient told me that his chronic neck pain had decreased by approximately 90 percent. He needed to see the chiropractor much less often and did not require frequent acupuncture treatments. He was delighted.

I explained to him that because of his dramatic response to vitamin D, it was a sign that he had had osteomalacia of his neck bones. Osteomalacia is adult rickets! With severe vitamin D deficiency, there is a defect in the bone-hardening process, characterized by a deep, gnawing pain in the muscles and bones.

After several months, we repeated the blood test to assess his vitamin D level, and indeed, his levels were now over 40 ng/ml.

The patient that I have just described to you was *me*. Because of my Sikh dress (which covers most of my body) and my fair skin and subsequent sun avoidance, my vitamin D level started out extremely low. In correcting it, my neck pain was basically eliminated. I had cured myself of osteomalacia!

Incidence of Vitamin D Deficiency

The statistics regarding vitamin D deficiency are startling. However, it is not my intention to strike fear into your heart but to present you with some facts. Vitamin D deficiency is reaching epidemic proportions, and it is affecting the current and long-term health of our children. But despite the alarming statistics, vitamin D deficiency is very simple to correct (and I will show you how I do that in Chapter 5).

Children and Vitamin D Deficiency

Children are spending an increasing amount of time indoors, and when they are outside, they are covered with sunscreen and protective clothing. This has increased the prevalence of vitamin D deficiency. Several research studies have gathered information about children's levels of vitamin D and reported a high incidence of deficiency.

In studies conducted in Maine and Massachusetts, 52 percent of African-American and Hispanic adolescents and 48 percent of white preadolescent girls were deficient in vitamin D. Another study conducted in the winter throughout the United States revealed that 42 percent of females aged 15 to 49 were deficient. The studies all showed these groups to have vitamin D blood levels of less than 20 ng/ml, which exposes them to a risk of osteomalacia. However, one Boston study showed that 24 percent of the girls tested during their annual physical had levels below 15 ng/ml, and 14 percent had levels below 8 ng/ml! European children are found to be at high risk for vitamin D deficiency because few foods are fortified with the vitamin. Even in sunny parts of the world such as India, Turkey, and Lebanon, between 30 and 50 percent of the children studied had deficient vitamin D levels (less than 20 ng/ml).

Infants who are breast-fed exclusively are at risk for vitamin D deficiency. Most human breast milk contains very little naturally occurring vitamin D, typically only about 20 IU of vitamin D per one liter. A breast-fed baby will not get sufficient vitamin D unless their mother has vitamin D levels of at least 30 ng/ml, and the baby will be better off if the nursing mother has a level of 40 ng/ml or higher. So if the mother is deficient and is not taking vitamin D supplements, then the breast-fed child will also be deficient. Although taking oral vitamin D is safe for infants, many who are breast-fed are not given any supplementation. As a result these children have blood levels of less than 20 ng/ml, which increases their risk for getting rickets. This explains why researchers are reporting a rise in the number of incidents of rickets in infants who are exclusively breast-fed. (See Chapter 5 for my recommendations.)

This leads us into a look at pregnant and nursing mothers.

Pregnant and Nursing Mothers and Vitamin D Deficiency

In a study of women giving birth—despite taking their prenatal vitamins with 400 IU of vitamin D—73 percent of the women were severely vitamin D deficient, and 80 percent of the babies had severe vitamin D deficiency at birth. Many of the mothers were taking a multivitamin with 400 IU of vitamin D and were also drinking vitamin D–fortified milk every day. Some of the women in these studies had severely deficient levels of 10 and 15 ng/ml.

Vitamin D penetrates a woman's milk in correlation with her own blood level, and a mother who takes 400 IU/day is still not able to raise the vitamin D level of her breast-feeding baby. However, mothers who take

4,000 IU/day can raise the blood levels of their babies to greater than 30 ng/ml.

A New York study showed that 69 percent of paired infants and mothers were vitamin D deficient. A Canadian study found that only 11 percent of women in their second trimester had adequate levels of vitamin D in their blood. Women who are breast-feeding may also be diminishing their own levels of vitamin D as they pass on their own stores of it to their babies.

Recommendations are now coming out for pregnant women to get their vitamin D level tested every three or four months during pregnancy, and that is what I do in my own practice.

Obesity and Vitamin D Deficiency

Because vitamin D is a fat-soluble vitamin, it is absorbed by, and stored in, fat cells. In people who are obese, there are more fat cells to collect the vitamin D that has been ingested or made from sun exposure. As a result, there is less vitamin D available to the kidneys and intestines and therefore less calcium available to maintain strong bones.

In a study published in the summer of 2008, blood levels of postmenopausal women living in the U.K. at 57 degrees north latitude were found to be on average 23 ng/ml in the fall, even though they are supposed to be at their highest at this time. In the spring, their levels were an average of 19 ng/ml. Researchers associated these low levels with bone loss and obesity and observed that the women in the study with the highest body mass index (BMI) had the lowest levels of vitamin D.

Michael Holick, M.D., Ph.D., has made a connection between people who are obese and vitamin D deficiency–related osteomalacia. He indicated that individuals who are obese and deficient in vitamin D might experience muscle weakness and pain. They may tend to exercise less because of the pain and weakness, which in turn can increase obesity. While more research is necessary in this area, Dr. Holick indicated that treating obese people for vitamin D deficiency could relieve the pain of osteomalacia and make way for them to increase their physical activity.

The Elderly and Vitamin D Deficiency

More than half of Americans over 65 are vitamin D deficient, putting them at greater risk for bone fractures. Elderly people, especially those who are shut-ins, are at high risk for vitamin D deficiency because they are not getting adequate exposure to the sun. As many as 30 percent of those who are over 60 years of age, even if they are living at lower latitudes (closer to the equator), have been shown to have insufficient levels of vitamin D in the winter (lower than 30 ng/ml). Up to 26 percent of elderly people living in higher latitudes have blood vitamin D levels of less than 30 ng/ml in the summer. Even if elderly people do get some sun exposure, their ability to metabolize vitamin D becomes less efficient as they age, as they have less vitamin D precursor in the skin. Compared to young people, elderly adults need up to four times more exposure to UVB rays to make adequate vitamin D. Older individuals may also tend to be even more sun scared and more likely to avoid exposure, therefore, decreasing their usable vitamin D levels.

Low levels of vitamin D in elderly people can cause osteoporosis and make existing osteoporosis worsen. As the U.S. population ages, researchers expect the number of osteoporosis-related fractures to increase from more than 2 million in 2005 to more than 3 million in 2025. The associated medical costs were estimated to have been $17 billion in 2005 and are projected to be more than $25 billion in 2025.

According to researchers, levels of vitamin D that are lower than 30 ng/ml have appeared to increase the risk of fractures in elderly people. Of great concern to my patients who have elderly parents is the fear of their parents falling and sustaining injury or fracture. As people age, they may lose muscle mass and strength, and this weakening can lead to an increased risk of falling. Researchers have estimated that by age 65, one in three people falls each year, and one in two falls each year by the age of 80. About 20 to 30 percent of those who fall sustain an injury, and at least 50 percent of those injuries are fractures.

Muscle performance in elderly people may also be affected by low levels of vitamin D. Researchers have discovered vitamin D receptors in the muscles, and insufficient levels of vitamin D (lower than 30 ng/ml) are associated with impaired performance in the lower extremities.

In subsequent chapters, I will discuss the heartening findings that researchers have made regarding vitamin D supplementation and its positive effects on falls, fractures, bone loss, and muscle performance in the elderly.

Others Who May Have Vitamin D Deficiency

As I have mentioned, vitamin D is fat soluble. People who have illnesses that prevent them from absorbing fat properly could be at risk for vitamin D deficiency. Individuals with diseases such as Crohn's disease and cystic fibrosis may be unable to absorb fat-soluble vitamin D properly. Those who have undergone gastric-bypass surgery may have a diminished ability to absorb fat and, therefore, vitamin D. If you have had liver or kidney failure, that could impair the ability of these organs to process vitamin D.

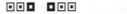

To sum up, with these incidence reports of vitamin D deficiency, it becomes clear that most people are at risk. As I have explained, even with the best intentions of raising your levels of vitamin D, you could still be deficient. Despite drinking milk, eating salmon, and taking a multivitamin, 32 percent of healthy people studied in Boston were found to have deficient levels of vitamin D. After 25 years of experience as an integrative-medicine doctor, I diagnosed myself with adult rickets! Believe me, anyone can be vitamin D deficient.

Now that you are familiar with the details of vitamin D deficiency, let us move on to the next chapter and examine what researchers are saying about the diseases and illnesses associated with vitamin D deficiency.

Chapter Four

ILLNESS, DISEASE, AND VITAMIN D DEFICIENCY

In my 30-year medical career, I have never seen a substance gain the media attention being afforded to vitamin D. Some have called it "vitamin D hype." The word *hype* means excessive, but it also implies that something is false or fabricated. My goal is to help you clarify the information presented in the scientific studies and present you with the facts—without hype. The following commentary simplifies vitamin D research on more than 20 diseases and conditions.

On June 10, 2008, the *Los Angeles Times* ran a story titled "Sunshine May Be Nature's Disease Fighter." The article reported that there was a sudden influx of research findings being released indicating that low vitamin D levels increase the risk of juvenile diabetes, breast cancer, and heart attack.

In the developed nations of the world, 60 to 70 percent of total mortality is attributed to diseases and conditions such as cancer, cardiovascular disease, and diabetes mellitus. In a review of 18 different vitamin D deficiency studies, it was found that people taking vitamin D were *less likely* to die from any cause while people not taking vitamin D supplementation were *more likely* to die.

This is the launching point for a discussion on the link between vitamin D and disease. In general terms, the experts are saying that if you are taking vitamin D, you are less likely to die from any health condition. In fact, one study indicated that vitamin D could increase longevity by 7 percent. This study specifically used a low dose (528 IU) and the trials were very short, but a noticeable increase was still observed.

Overwhelming statistics have shown that most people who have a serious disease also have vitamin D deficiency or were deficient in the past. Many studies have determined that vitamin D may provide protection from illnesses ranging from the common cold to cancer.

Children's diseases such as autism, asthma, and juvenile diabetes have become pervasive in the years that we have been told to avoid the sun; and vitamin D deficiency is suspected to be connected with these diseases. In regard to vitamin D and disease, Robert Heaney, M.D., researcher and professor of medicine at Creighton University, has said, "We don't really know what the status of chronic disease is in the North American population until we normalize vitamin D status."

Long-Latency Deficiency Diseases

Other than osteomalacia and rickets, all the diseases associated with vitamin D deficiency are what doctors call "Long-Latency Deficiency Diseases."

In 2003, Dr. Heaney published a paper titled "Long-Latency Deficiency Disease." In it, he discussed how most national nutritional policies (such as the RDA) have been primarily oriented toward just preventing a short-latency deficiency disease. In the case of vitamin D, such a short-latency disease would be rickets. And in the case of vitamin C, it would be scurvy.

"Short latency" refers to the relatively short length of time it takes for symptoms—such as musculoskeletal pain, or illnesses like osteomalacia or rickets—to show up when a person is deprived of a nutrient. "Long latency" refers to the many years it often takes for some types of diseases to present themselves. Three long-latency disorders that afflict society today include cancer, cardiovascular disease, and central nervous system degeneration.

Dr. Heaney goes on to talk about how most nutrient recommendations are solely based on the prevention of short-latency disease. It is then taken for granted that if the intake of a particular nutrient is sufficient to prevent the short-latency illness, then it must also be sufficient for all of the functioning in our body.

However, doses that prevent the short-term problem are now found to be inadequate for optimizing some of the other important functions of that nutrient over the long term. We are finding that long-term inadequate intakes of several nutrients, including vitamin D, are contributing to several of the major chronic diseases that affect the populations of all industrialized nations.

Sometimes these long-latency deficiency diseases come about by the same biochemical mechanism that produces a short-latency disease. However, in the case of most of the diseases that have been recently associated with vitamin D deficiency, additional biochemical mechanisms appear to be involved and may require years for the subsequent disease to be clinically recognizable.

In addition, as I have mentioned, the intake of the nutrient required to prevent many of the long-latency disorders is usually higher than that required to prevent the short-latency diseases. In other words, you may need to take more vitamin D to help prevent cancer than you need to take to help prevent osteomalacia. Therefore, recommendations that are based solely on preventing the short-latency disease cannot necessarily be applied to the long-latency nutritional deficiency diseases.

In a paper published in 2002, Dr. William B. Grant, the director of the Sunlight, Nutrition, and Health Research Center, estimated that as much as 20 percent of breast-cancer cases in Europe were a result of vitamin D deficiency. To the degree that this conclusion is correct, breast cancer would represent a long-latency deficiency disorder that involves an entirely different mechanism from that of rickets, the classical vitamin D deficiency disease.

The impact of vitamin D has such sweeping ramifications that we will not know the true status of disease until we address vitamin D deficiency. The vitamin D expert Dr. Cedric Garland gave his views of the implications of correcting worldwide vitamin D deficiency: "The first thing we'd see is a reduction by 80 percent in the incidence of Type 1 diabetes. The next thing we'd see is a reduction by about 75 percent of all invasive cancers combined, as well as similar reductions in colon cancer and breast cancer, and probably about a 25 percent reduction in ovarian cancer."

Understanding the Different Research Methods

The most important type of research to a medical doctor like me is a *prospective* study. Using this method, researchers identify participants for their study, decide in advance what they are going to be doing and watching for, and follow the participants forward through time. This establishes a relationship between the variables (vitamin D) and the outcome (the effect of vitamin D on the illness).

Most of the studies discussed in this book showing an association between vitamin D deficiency and a particular disease are not prospective studies; rather, they are *epidemiological* or they are "open" trials. *Epidemiological* studies go back in time and examine data in order to find an association between two or more variables; and then scientists report on what they have discovered. Sometimes these are called *retrospective studies* because they look back in time. *"Open" trials* are where patients and doctors know what each patient is taking, and their results are observed.

The authors of these latter types of studies will often look at the data in many ways, using numerous statistical methods to rule out other causes for the results they are observing. These are the types of trials that have been done for virtually every disease that is associated with vitamin D deficiency, other than bone disease and fractures.

The true gold standard in medicine and science is known as the *prospective randomized placebo-controlled trial.* Let us look at what this means: *Prospective,* as I have just explained, means that researchers planned the study from the beginning and will be looking forward with the interventions given to patients. *Randomized* means that patients are randomly put into one of two groups. And *placebo controlled* signifies that one of the groups receives a placebo or "dummy" pill of inert substances, and the other group is given the actual substance being tested (in this case, vitamin D).

These patients are then followed over the ensuing period of time, usually years. Neither the doctors who are involved with the patients nor the patients themselves know whether they are getting the placebo or the vitamin D. At the end of the duration of the study, the researchers evaluate whether taking vitamin D had any effect on the disease or illness. Of course, this is a simplified explanation of a very complex and exact process. Given ethical concerns of not giving *any* vitamin D, these days the placebo group is usually given a lower dose of vitamin D rather than none at all.

Prospective randomized-controlled trials (RCTs) are currently being planned for many aspects of vitamin D treatment. However, by their very nature, the results will not be available for many years, maybe even a decade.

In the next section, I am going to simplify some of the complex scientific research that has been conducted in support of this investigation of the role that vitamin D plays in cancer. Then in Section II, I will review the research that shows the connection of vitamin D to many other illnesses.

SECTION I—VITAMIN D AND CANCER

Researchers in the United States have estimated that every year, 60,000 premature deaths from cancer are caused by insufficient levels of vitamin D. This translates into 10 percent of total cancer deaths being attributed to insufficient vitamin D. Applying the statistics to Canadian cancer deaths, 7,000 deaths can be attributed to low vitamin D levels.

Is it really possible that a simple substance like vitamin D could provide protection from something as complex as cancer? It may seem like an outlandish claim, but I assure you that researchers have been diligent in carrying out studies and reviews to advance the understanding of the relationship between vitamin D and cancer. In fact, the information in these studies was so compelling to me that I had to write this book!

We Have a Prospective
Study on Vitamin D and Cancer!

I am happy to say that a major prospective study was recently released, published in 2007 by *The American Journal of Clinical Nutrition*. The study set out to determine whether vitamin D and/or calcium had a preventive effect on non–skin cancer. In addition to being a prospective study, lead author Dr. Joan M. Lappe and her colleagues created a randomized, double-blind, placebo-controlled trial. These terms mean that neither the randomly selected participants (postmenopausal women) nor the researchers knew what intervention participants were getting (vitamin D and/or calcium, or a placebo). In this study, the placebo group got only a "dummy" pill with neither vitamin D nor calcium.

This is the first prospective study to provide evidence that vitamin D provides protection against cancer in postmenopausal women. And it is the first study that allows me to safely and confidently say to my patients that vitamin D helps protect them against cancer! This is good news—even if you are not a postmenopausal woman. I expect that these results will fully transfer to women and men of all ages.

While I remain cautious, because many more prospective studies with different groups of people need to be conducted to solidify these findings, I am confident in the recommendations I am making to my patients to optimize their vitamin D levels.

This groundbreaking study was conducted in Nebraska on 403 postmenopausal women over a period of four years. The researchers reported that the women who received 1,100 IU of vitamin D and 1,000 mg (milligrams) of calcium per day for four years reduced their risk of developing cancer of any kind by 60 percent compared to those women who received a placebo.

During the first year of the study, some women developed cancer, and the researchers theorized that their cancers likely had been developing before the launch of the study. When they adjusted the statistics, removing the first year of the study, the results were even more dramatic. Those postmenopausal women taking calcium and vitamin D had a reduced risk of any kind of cancer of 77 percent.

The researchers acknowledged that their data showing that improving vitamin D levels reduced all cancer risk was consistent with the epidemiological and observational studies conducted over the years. Calcium alone had been found to reduce all cancers by 47 percent compared to placebo, but the results for the vitamin D–calcium combination were stunning.

Another finding of the same study indicated that for every 10 ng/ml increase in blood levels of vitamin D, the relative risk of cancer dropped by 35 percent. This is easily done, too. Michael Holick, M.D., Ph.D., has indicated that 1,000 IU of vitamin D per day, taken for several months, raises the blood level by 10 ng/ml.

Many researchers wonder if the avoidance of sun because of fear of skin cancer is worth the increased risk of and mortality from internal cancers.

The First Significant Link Between Vitamin D and Cancer

Investigation into the vitamin D and sun-exposure link to cancer began in 1980, when researchers Cedric and Frank Garland studied cancer mortality rates in the United States. They mapped the incidence of deaths from colon cancer and discovered that the lowest colon-cancer rates were in the southwestern states, and the highest rates were in the northeastern states. This work launched the connection between the sun and cancer. Subsequent studies showed similar geographical distribution of all kinds of cancers.

This type of study is called an epidemiological study, and it reviews the distribution and incidence of disease in different populations. Studies looking at latitude and its effect on vitamin D levels, cancer, and illness are epidemiological. As you will see, these studies provide evidence that the occurrence of many illnesses and diseases are not random.

Epidemiological studies allow scientists to make links between vitamin D and cancer, but they are not the "gold standard" that orthodox medicine requires to determine that vitamin D prevents cancer. However, these studies are important and give us an understanding of the possible relationship between vitamin D and cancer or illnesses, yet they do not provide the incontrovertible evidence necessary for all medical doctors to start recommending vitamin D.

Retrospective studies, as I have mentioned, look back on data that has already been gathered and seek to answer questions of the present time. For example, the Nurses' Health Study began in 1976 with 122,000 nurses aged 30 to 55 who completed a health questionnaire. In 1989 and 1990, 33,000 blood samples were taken, and another 18,700 were taken between 2000 and 2001. These blood samples were frozen and stored for future measurements. In this study, the health status of these nurses is still being followed to this day.

Current vitamin D researchers are able to take those test tubes out of the freezer from up to 20 years ago and analyze them for the vitamin D levels that were present at the time the blood was drawn. At the onset of the Nurses' Health Study, the association between vitamin D levels and disease had not yet been made.

With the current excitement about vitamin D, researchers are able to retrospectively look at vitamin

D levels in those blood samples and analyze the incidence of illness and cancer that have already occurred in this group of women. While we cannot draw final conclusions from these kinds of studies, the evidence of the link between vitamin D deficiency and illness has become quite compelling over the years.

Many retrospective and/or epidemiological studies have confirmed that people living at higher latitudes— north of 35 degrees latitude—are at a higher risk for developing cancer and are more likely to die from cancer than people living at lower latitudes. Seasonal studies have shown that people diagnosed with cancer (colon, breast, and prostate) in the summer or the fall had a better chance of survival than those diagnosed with cancer in the winter or spring. This was attributed to the likelihood that the patients had higher levels of vitamin D during these times of the year.

How Might Vitamin D Affect Cancer?

Dr. Lappe and colleagues indicated that the way vitamin D may protect against cancer is still being defined, but the current understanding shows that high levels of vitamin D may enhance the regulation of apoptosis, cell differentiation, and cell proliferation. The following is a summary of what the top researchers are saying about the mechanisms by which vitamin D may be protecting us from cancer.

Apoptosis. Apoptosis is a normal process where cells die off. Cells die as a natural course when they become compromised in some way so that newer, healthier cells can take their place. Apoptosis is also called programmed cell death. Cancer cells lose this ability, which causes them to grow uncontrollably. Vitamin D helps make cells that are turning cancerous die when they are supposed to.

Cell differentiation. Normal cells evolve and take on specialized jobs. For example, cells in an embryo become more specialized and evolve to develop into specific tissues and organs. Eventually, normal cells differentiate until they can no longer divide, and they stop growing when they have reached maturity. Cancer cells lose their ability to differentiate and, therefore, do not stop growing. They can reproduce haphazardly and quickly. Vitamin D helps make cancer cells differentiate and forces them to specialize into the types of cells within an organ that they are supposed to become.

Cellular proliferation. The growth and division of cells in the body is known as proliferation. The genes that control cellular proliferation are affected by vitamin D. If vitamin D levels are low, the ability of genes to affect proliferation is impaired.

Regulating cell growth. Vitamin D prevents angiogenesis, which is the formation and differentiation of blood vessels. Cancer cells create new blood vessels so the cancer can grow. Vitamin D impacts the genes that control angiogenesis, blocking cancer cells from creating new blood vessels (so they cannot keep growing).

Reduction of metastasis. Metastasis is the ability of a cancer cell to enter the bloodstream and travel to other parts of the body and invade normal, healthy tissues. Animal studies have indicated that vitamin D may inhibit the ability of cancer cells to spread in this way.

When vitamin D finishes its work in the cells, it destroys itself and does not release any activated vitamin D into the bloodstream or have any further effect on calcium metabolism.

Once you understand the mechanisms by which vitamin D protects the cells, you can see why researchers contend that a vitamin D deficiency is a risk factor for cancer. Knowing these interactions also gives insights into one reason why cancer may occur in otherwise healthy people. Further it allows you to understand why the authors of many of the research studies on cancer and vitamin D are calling for the government to increase the RDA guidelines for vitamin D.

I feel confident in these new higher dose recommendations when I reflect on my own practice—my experience mirrors exactly what these researchers have found. I too have seen many people develop cancer without having any of the risk factors commonly associated with it. Slim, healthy men and women who maintain nutritious diets and who never smoke cigarettes or consume alcohol get cancer, too. Typically these patients, in my practice, have very low vitamin D levels.

Vitamin D has been linked to the reduction of risk of 17 different types of cancer.

The vitamin D advocates have lots of credible science to fall back on. Studies link vitamin D deficiency with the following types of cancer: colon, breast, prostate, bladder, esophageal, gastric, ovarian, rectal, renal, uterine, cervical, gall bladder, laryngeal, oral, pancreatic, and non-Hodgkin's and Hodgkin's lymphomas. I will now discuss some of these.

Breast Cancer

According to recent estimates by the American Cancer Society (ACS), breast cancer is the second-leading cause of cancer deaths in women in the United States. Rates of breast cancer are higher in white women after the age of 40 but higher in black women before the age of 40. Black women are more likely to die from breast cancer at any age.

Breast tissue has vitamin D receptors so if there is sufficient vitamin D available, it can be activated in the breast. This sets up a series of events in the breast—specifically, the presence of activated vitamin D is believed to help protect cells from cancer, help repair cells that may be mutating with cancer, and help slow the proliferation of cancer cells that may be present. Cancer cells can be more prone to die when vitamin D assists in maintaining the cells' function of apoptosis. Activated vitamin D is also believed to interfere with tumors as they build blood vessels to feed themselves, thus starving the tumors.

Women who have a vitamin D blood level of less than 20 ng/ml may have a higher incidence of breast cancer by up to 50 percent. Research in human and animal studies suggests that inadequate exposure to vitamin D during puberty could affect normal breast development. Despite these findings, the American

Cancer Society published a booklet on breast cancer in 2007 that makes no mention of vitamin D deficiency and its relationship to the disease. In my opinion, optimizing vitamin D levels is a healthy option for people who have been told that they are at risk for developing breast cancer.

A 1999 study was the first to link breast cancer with sun exposure, concluding that the sun and vitamin D could potentially reduce the risk of breast cancer. By combining sun exposure, supplements, and vitamin D–rich food, the authors of the study estimated that between 70,000 and 150,000 new cases of breast cancer could be prevented per year, and that up to 37,500 deaths from breast cancer could be averted each year.

In another study published in 2008, researchers measured the vitamin D levels of 103 premenopausal women from the northeastern United States when they were newly diagnosed with breast cancer, and they found that 84 percent of the women were deficient in vitamin D (median levels of 15 ng/ml). Fewer women who were white had vitamin D deficiency (78 percent) than women who were black (90 percent) or Hispanic (91 percent).

For one year, the women were given the RDA of vitamin D (400 IU/day). When tested again, only 10 percent of the white and Hispanic women had achieved sufficient levels of vitamin D (above 30 ng/ml). None of the black women had increased their levels of vitamin D to sufficiency. The study concluded that the current RDA of vitamin D was insufficient to raise levels to 30 ng/ml in women with breast cancer.

Goodwin's Breast Cancer and Vitamin D Study

I believe that the most important recent study showing the association between breast cancer and vitamin D was by Dr. Pamela Goodwin and her associates and reported in spring 2008 when it caused quite a stir in the media. This was a retrospective study conducted in Toronto, Canada, where the researchers looked back at blood that had been taken from 512 women when they were diagnosed with breast cancer between 1989 and 1995. They followed the women on average for over 11 years.

In retrospect, the researchers saw that a startling 76 percent of the women in the study had insufficient or deficient levels of vitamin D when they were initially diagnosed with breast cancer. Only 24 percent had sufficient levels of vitamin D at the time of diagnosis.

The researchers made the association that the women who had had deficient levels at the time they were diagnosed were 73 percent more likely to die from breast cancer than those who had had sufficient levels of vitamin D at the time of diagnosis. Furthermore, women with deficient levels at the time of diagnosis were almost twice as likely to have a recurrence or spread of the cancer. However, women who started with normal levels of vitamin D in their blood had an 83 percent chance of surviving without further spread of cancer over the course of the study. To quote the conclusion of the study: "Vitamin D deficiency is common at breast cancer diagnosis and is associated with poor prognosis."

In My Opinion . . .

My wife and I had the privilege of hearing a vitamin D expert discussing this study on the radio. In the interview, this expert advised women with the diagnosis of breast cancer *against* taking vitamin D until prospective randomized-controlled trials could be run.

At a staff conference, I presented this startling information about the association between vitamin D and breast-cancer prognosis to my mostly female staff. I explained that this study was only associating higher vitamin D with a better prognosis, but that it did not actually prove that taking vitamin D would have any benefit.

My entire staff looked at me as if I were crazy. It was obvious to them that taking some vitamin D, which is inexpensive and harmless, would in no way hurt them and might significantly benefit them. I, too, disagree with the expert who was interviewed on the radio. I realize that large, randomized-controlled trials that measure the benefit of vitamin D in the treatment and prevention of illness and disease must be run. Until then, we cannot advertise with certainty that taking vitamin D will help protect people against cancer and the other diseases that I am describing in this book. However, it is going to take many years, even a decade, to have conclusive results.

Given all the knowledge we have today and the strong associations made by most experts in the field, what harm is it for a person to take 2,000 IU/day when vitamin D is so readily available and inexpensive? Certainly it will do no harm (as I will illustrate in the following chapter that up to 10,000 IU/day is probably safe), and in light of all the studies, it will certainly help optimize the functioning of vitamin D in a person's body.

The lack of randomized-controlled trials (RCT) may be an argument for a "by the book" doctor to refrain from using vitamin D for the purpose of helping a woman with her breast cancer. But as John Cannell, M.D., and others contend in the January 2008 issue of *Expert Opinion Pharmacotherapy:*

Is that an argument not to diagnose and treat vitamin D deficiency? If human RCTs exist showing cigarette smoking is dangerous, the authors have yet to locate them. Instead, the compelling evidence for the dangerousness of smoking exists in convincing epidemiological data and the demonstration of a mechanism of action. The same is true for vitamin D, although the diseases linked to vitamin D deficiency outnumber those linked to cigarette smoking . . . and activated vitamin D, a secosteroid, has as many mechanisms of actions as genes it targets. Some would also argue that the quantity and quality of the epidemiological data for vitamin D is approaching that which existed for cigarette smoking when governments and medical bodies first acted.

Increased Risk of Breast Cancer with Lower Vitamin D Levels

According to another paper presented by a large group of vitamin D researchers (Garland, Gorham, and Mohr, among others), insufficient vitamin D from the sun or supplements is associated with a higher risk of developing breast cancer.

The team of researchers analyzed the pooled data collected from two studies that associated breast-cancer risk with vitamin D levels. In both studies, the risk was lower in women who had higher levels of vitamin D. Furthermore, the odds of developing breast cancer decreased as the daily dose and corresponding blood levels of vitamin D increased.

It was projected that a vitamin D blood level of approximately 52 ng/ml would reduce the risk of breast cancer by 50 percent from the risk that is present when vitamin D blood levels are less than 13 ng/ml. To achieve this level of 25D, an estimated daily dose of 4,000 IU of vitamin D was recommended either from supplements or sun exposure or a combination of both.

The researchers also estimated the number of U.S. breast-cancer cases that could potentially be prevented if women maintained certain blood levels of vitamin D. For example, at levels of 32 ng/ml, it was projected that 66,000 new cases of breast cancer per year could be prevented, whereas vitamin D levels of 52 ng/ml could potentially prevent 107,000 new cases of breast cancer per year.

In other words, according to Garland and his colleagues, based on the existing studies, they project that women who have vitamin D levels of about 52 ng/ml would have 50 percent less risk of getting breast cancer than women with vitamin D levels below 13 ng/ml. This is a major difference and certainly gives us a lot to think about.

Given a choice, I know that my female staff members, family, and friends would prefer to raise their vitamin D levels to 52 ng/ml.

A Vitamin D and Breast-Cancer Case

Susan is a 52-year-old woman with metastatic breast cancer. She consulted with me, as many breast-cancer patients do, for "immune support." She was getting ongoing chemotherapy and felt exhausted and nauseated most of the time.

I was hopeful that with acupuncture and some supportive herbs, her nausea could improve. As is my routine, I also checked her vitamin D level, which was only 8 ng/ml, alerting me to her severe deficiency. I told Susan that I wanted to start her on a relatively high dose of vitamin D to try to get her numbers up to 50 ng/ml, in light of her metastatic breast cancer. She thanked me very much for the visit, but I did not hear back from her.

Just recently, over a year later, Susan returned to my office very chagrined. She brought her most recent scans that showed the metastases had been spreading through her body, especially to her bones. I remembered that I had informed her about vitamin D and was hopeful that it might help her retard the progression of the disease. I asked her whether she started taking a vitamin D supplement, and to my disappointment, she replied that her oncologist had said, "Vitamins aren't going to help you, and too much vitamin D can be toxic. Don't take it."

I gave Susan a plethora of articles to take back to her oncologist and have now encouraged her to take a high dose of vitamin D. I plan to track her blood level until she reaches an optimal level, and I continue to be hopeful for her prognosis.

In my practice, I give vitamin D to all my many breast-cancer patients, and I keep their blood levels optimized.

Several researchers question the logic behind sun avoidance to prevent skin cancer when other serious internal cancers are killing more people. Vitamin D expert Dr. Michael Holick did the math. For every person who dies from skin cancer (attributed to overexposure to the sun), 55 women die from breast cancer (which has a relationship with underexposure to the sun).

Vitamin D and Lung Cancer

According to recent estimates by the American Cancer Society (ACS), lung cancer is the leading cause of cancer death in men and women in the United States. Non-small-cell lung cancer is the most common type, affecting 85 to 90 percent of those diagnosed with the disease. At the time of this writing, there was no mention in the ACS's current online literature of vitamin D or UVB deficiency as risk factors for developing lung cancer. The organization states that: "Some people who get lung cancer do not have any known risk factors."

One study found that lung-cancer patients who had high sun exposure or had a high intake of vitamin D had three times the survival rate of lung-cancer patients with lower vitamin D levels. A 2008 study published in the *Journal of Epidemiology and Community Health* revealed that increased incidence of lung cancer was associated with low levels of UVB sunlight in 111 countries.

In another study, patients with non-small-cell lung cancer who had the highest levels of vitamin D were twice as likely to avoid recurrence as people with the lowest levels of vitamin D. The researchers reported that untreated vitamin D deficiency put lung-cancer patients at risk for earlier death.

Researchers in Norway reviewed the data associated with cases of lung cancer (more than 15,000) reported between 1964 and 2000. From their research, they concluded that high levels of vitamin D from the sun were associated with a better prognosis for patients diagnosed with lung cancer. The Nordic countries are between 50 and 71 degrees latitude, making it impossible for people to produce vitamin D from the sun during the winter months. They found that vitamin D levels were up to 120 percent higher in the summer than in the winter, which may help explain why young men diagnosed with lung cancer in the autumn had a better prognosis than those diagnosed in the winter.

Vitamin D and Colon Cancer

According to the most recent estimates by the American Cancer Society, colorectal cancer is the third-leading cause of cancer death in the United States. Approximately, 108,070 new cases of colon cancer and 40,740 new cases of rectal cancer will be diagnosed in 2008. The ACS also states that "African Americans have the highest colorectal cancer incidence and mortality rates of all racial groups in the United States. The reason for this is not yet understood."

Prospective and retrospective studies determined that low vitamin D levels (below 20 ng/ml) were associated with a 20 to 50 percent increased risk of colon cancer (also prostate and breast cancers) as well as with a risk for higher mortality from these cancers. Another meta-analysis of cancer studies estimated that vitamin D blood levels of approximately 33 ng/ml were associated with an estimated 50 percent lower risk for colon cancer compared to those with levels of 12 ng/ml.

Another retrospective study that I have mentioned, the Nurses' Health Study (with over 32,000 patients), showed that the likelihood of getting colon cancer was inversely associated with vitamin D blood levels. Nurses whose blood levels of vitamin D were higher than 39 ng/ml had a 47 percent reduction in the likelihood of getting colon cancer compared to those with a blood level of 16 ng/ml.

Patients in The Women's Health Initiative Study (retrospective), who at the start of the study had a vitamin D level of less than 12 ng/ml, experienced a 253 percent increase in the risk of colon cancer over a period of eight years. According to Dr. Michael Holick in the May 25, 2006, issue of the *New England Journal of Medicine*, "Virtually all the subjects in the study had vitamin D insufficiency . . . both at the beginning and at the end of the trial. . . . These women needed more vitamin D."

A prospective study in over 1,900 men showed a 47 percent reduction in relative likelihood of getting colon cancer with an intake of 230 to 650 IU/day compared to taking between 6 and 94 IU/day of vitamin D.

In a Boston study published in 2008, a team of researchers led by Dr. Kimmie Ng and Dr. Charles Fuchs selected data on 304 patients who had been diagnosed with colon cancer between 1991 and 2002. The patients' health was followed until they died or until 2005, whichever came first. The team found that the patients with the highest levels of vitamin D were 48 percent less likely to die from colon cancer or any other cause when compared to the patients who had the lowest vitamin D levels. For colon cancer alone, the patients with the highest vitamin D levels were 39 percent less likely to die compared with those with the lowest vitamin D levels. In other words, the higher the levels of vitamin D in the system two years before a colon-cancer diagnosis, the higher the rates of survival of the patients during follow-up.

About this study, Dr. Holick commented: "This finding is outstanding. It is consistent with dozens and dozens of observations that have been made in the past decade." More research in this area needs to be done in the form of prospective studies before we can say for sure that vitamin D prevents colon cancer. However, these studies do provide us with information that speaks for itself and cannot be ignored.

Vitamin D and Prostate Cancer

In 2008, approximately 186,320 new cases of prostate cancer are expected to be diagnosed in the United States according to the ACS. About one man in six will be diagnosed with prostate cancer during his lifetime, and more African-American men are diagnosed with prostate cancer than any other race. The reason why prostate cancer affects a disproportionate number of African-American men is unknown.

A retrospective study showed that the average age of men who developed prostate cancer was three to five years later in men who had sun exposure throughout their lives. Another interesting study showed that men who had high sun exposure as a youth were less likely to develop prostate cancer in adulthood.

Like most tissues and cells in the body, the prostate has vitamin D receptors—activated vitamin D is manufactured on-site. Vitamin D in the prostate protects healthy prostate cells and tells cells to die on time so that they are less likely to grow into cancer.

According to one study, men with metastatic prostate cancer who were given 2,000 IU of vitamin D daily for 21 months had up to a 50 percent reduction in their PSA (prostate-specific antigen) levels. With vitamin D supplementation, PSA counts did not accelerate as quickly.

Dr. Michael Holick commented on the overwhelming evidence linking sun avoidance with incidences of prostate cancer. He indicated that for every one man who dies from skin cancer, which is probably associated with overexposure to the sun, 55 to 60 men die of prostate cancer, which is probably related to a lack of sun exposure and low vitamin D.

The results of an epidemiological study published in 2004 found inconsistencies in the data reviewed of prostate cancer cases in Nordic men. It appeared that vitamin D levels below 19 ng/ml and levels above 80 ng/ml were both associated with increased prostate cancer risk. The authors indicated that low levels may impair the ability of the tissue to control cell proliferation, while high vitamin D levels may be associated with vitamin D resistance.

My Reflections on Vitamin D and Cancer

Vitamin D deficiency is connected with 17 different varieties of cancer, and credible scientific studies conducted by the country's foremost vitamin D experts show that optimizing a cancer patient's vitamin D level is an essential prerequisite for good oncology care. I agree with doctors of integrative medicine who define "optimal" as between 40 to 70 ng/ml, based on my own clinical practice.

I see new patients who have cancer on a regular basis. It is my great sorrow to report that thus far, I have yet to encounter a cancer patient who has had a vitamin D test done by their oncologist or their regular physician. Yet almost every cancer patient I see is significantly deficient at the first measurement. As Dr. Cannell has suggested (in the journal *Expert Opinion*

Pharmacotherapy), I unfortunately envision a time in the future when lawsuits against physicians begin to appear claiming that doctors were negligent in *not* diagnosing and treating vitamin D deficiency in cancer patients. I would expect that unless the mainstream medical community acknowledges the connection between vitamin D and cancer, and unless oncologists recognize the importance of vitamin D deficiency, these types of malpractice suits could become very common.

This does not have to be the way of the future! Further, cancer rates are not predestined to rise year after year. As you have seen in the research I have presented, simply modifying our behaviors slightly can have a huge impact on our health.

It is my sincere hope that doctors and patients will take this research to heart so that we may use our time helping patients to get well and stay well. This is why I have shared all this with you.

SECTION II—VITAMIN D AND OTHER DISEASES AND ILLNESSES

We have finished discussing the relationship between vitamin D and cancer. Now we will review the connection between vitamin D and many other diseases and illnesses in modern society.

Vitamin D and Cardiovascular Health

Cardiovascular disease (CVD) includes hypertension (high blood pressure), coronary heart disease, heart failure, and stroke. According to the American Heart Association, one in three—or 80,700,000 people—have at least one form of CVD, with high blood pressure having the highest rates, affecting 73,000,000 Americans.

Risk factors that impact cardiovascular health include smoking, poor diet, lack of exercise, obesity, diabetes, and high cholesterol. At the time of this writing, the American Heart Association Website made no mention of vitamin D deficiency being a risk factor for CVD.

Incidences of CVD are reported to be significantly higher at higher latitudes where there is less access to healthy sun exposure. More people die from heart disease in the winter than in the summer when sun exposure is more easily attained.

The Health Professionals' Follow-Up Study

Earlier in the book, I talked about prospective studies and how they are so important to medical science in general, and my medical practice in particular because they provide me with credible evidence that a substance like vitamin D can have a positive impact on the health of my patients. In 2008 an important prospective study was published looking at vitamin D and the risk of heart attack.

The famous Health Professionals Follow-Up Study, led by Edward Giovannucci, M.D., collected blood samples from more than 51,000 male health professionals who were between the ages of 40 and 75 in 1986. The participants also completed a health questionnaire every two years. In addition, another blood sample was taken from more than 18,000 men between 1993 and 1995. Vitamin D levels were subsequently tested. At the time of this blood collection, none of the men had had a diagnosis of cardiovascular disease before 1994. Of the men participating in the study, only 23 percent had vitamin D levels above 30 ng/ml. This low percentage is typical of many populations in the world, and it is even lower in subpopulations of elderly or dark-skinned individuals.

In the ten years that followed (1994–2004), 454 of the men experienced non-fatal heart attacks or fatal coronary heart disease. They were compared with 900 men who had not had heart attacks during the time of the study.

What researchers found was that men who were deficient in vitamin D (with levels below 15 ng/ml) were 242 percent more likely to have a heart attack compared to men who had levels of at least 30 ng/ml. Their risk of heart attack was more than double the risk of their counterparts with higher vitamin D levels!

To determine the extent to which other factors affected heart attack in the participants, the researchers took into account other known risk factors associated with heart disease, such as family history of heart attack, body mass index, alcohol consumption, physical activity, history of diabetes mellitus and high blood pressure, ethnicity, region, omega-3 fatty acid intake, HDL and LDL (high- and low-density lipoprotein) cholesterol levels, and triglyceride levels.

After they removed all of the additional variables, they found that men who were deficient in vitamin D *still* had a 209 percent higher risk for heart attack than men with levels of at least 30 ng/ml. What this means is that even if there were other reasons why the men were more prone to having heart attacks, the lack of vitamin D in their bloodstream still doubled their risk. Furthermore, men whose vitamin D levels were between 22 and 29 ng/ml were still at a heightened risk

(160 percent) for heart attack compared to those with levels of 30 ng/ml or more.

Researchers broke the statistics down even more. The patients whose vitamin D levels were over 17 ng/ml had 30 percent of the risk of the patients whose blood levels were less than 10 ng/ml. This means that patients with vitamin D levels of less than 10 ng/ml had 70 percent more risk of having a heart attack than those with levels over 17 ng/ml. For each increase of 1 ng/ml in vitamin D blood levels, the risk of having a heart attack fell by 2 percent.

There was also an association suggested by the researchers that the patients with low vitamin D may be at risk for fatal heart attacks. The number of cases involved was too small to draw a definite conclusion, but it is worth mentioning here. This prospective study certainly shows that low levels of vitamin D are associated with a higher risk of heart attack.

It is significant to note that the vitamin D levels the researchers investigated were only 30 ng/ml, not what I believe to be optimal levels of 40 ng/ml or more. According to current standards held by integrative-medicine doctors, 30 ng/ml is considered to be a less than optimal level of blood vitamin D. Given the amazing results with 30 ng/ml cutting heart attack risk in half, I cannot help but wonder what effect optimal blood levels might have on heart-attack risk.

What Vitamin D Might Be Doing for the Heart

With respect to heart disease and all cardiovascular disease, vitamin D deficiency has been found to affect the muscle lining of the blood vessels and contribute to inflammation, as well as calcification of the vascular wall. It also affects the central part of the endocrine system that controls blood pressure. All of these factors affect the risk for heart disease and specifically heart attack.

Other Studies on Vitamin D and Heart Health

High blood pressure, the most common form of cardiovascular disease, improves when patients are exposed to UVB rays. Patients with hypertension were exposed to UVB rays three times a week for three months. The vitamin D levels in their blood increased by 180 percent, and their blood pressure normalized.

A 1999 randomized-controlled trial (RCT) measured participants' blood pressure after UVB tanning-bed exposure, and vitamin D blood levels were elevated by 162 percent, reducing systolic and diastolic blood pressure by six points each.

In the Health Professionals Follow-up Study as well as the Nurses' Health Study, men and women with vitamin D levels below 15 ng/ml were three times more likely to have a new diagnosis of high blood pressure/hypertension in the four years of follow-up, compared to those participants who had vitamin D levels greater than 30 ng/ml. The NHANES III (the National Health and Nutrition Examination Survey, which is compiled by the CDC) also showed an inverse association between vitamin D levels and blood pressure.

Several studies have connected low levels of vitamin D with other aspects of impaired cardiovascular health, including peripheral arterial disease, which is associated with reduced blood flow in the legs. Peripheral arterial disease is 64 percent more common in people who have low levels of vitamin D. Furthermore, the risk for this disease increased by 29 percent with every drop of 10 ng/ml in vitamin D levels in the blood.

Vitamin D levels in the patients with congestive heart failure were up to 50 percent lower than in people with healthy hearts. The participants with the worst cases of congestive heart failure had the lowest vitamin D levels as well as impaired calcium metabolism.

Researchers have identified that there are vitamin D receptors in the cells of the blood vessels. Vitamin D relaxes the blood vessels and reduces blood pressure. As reported in the journal *Circulation,* the Framingham Heart Study followed cases of 1,700 adults who did *not* have a history of cardiovascular disease over a period of five years. Of these volunteers, 120 had a cardiovascular event, which may have included the new onset of cardiac chest pain (angina), heart attacks, heart failure, strokes, and leg pain due to inadequate blood supply. The patients who had high blood pressure with the lowest levels of vitamin D had twice as many serious cardiovascular events compared to those with high blood pressure and the highest blood levels of vitamin D.

Another study concluded that because vitamin D has anti-inflammatory properties, it may be beneficial for people with congestive heart failure. The same study found that elevated parathyroid hormone (PTH), which is suppressed by vitamin D, may impair heart function.

Vitamin D and Bone Health—Osteoporosis

The National Osteoporosis Foundation in the U.S. measured the prevalence of osteoporosis and low bone mass based on numbers from the census of 2000. They calculated that approximately 55 percent of male and female Americans (44 million) over the age of 50 have either osteoporosis or low bone mass (osteopenia). It is estimated that this number will grow to 52 million by the year 2010 and to 61 million by 2020. In 2002, approximately 10 million people had the disease, and these numbers are increasing. By 2010, it is expected that 12 million people will have the disease, and 14 million will have it by the year 2020 unless an intervention is conducted. Approximately 80 percent of those with osteoporosis are women.

About 33 percent of women between 60 and 70 years old have osteoporosis, and 66 percent of women who are 80 and older have it. More than half the women who are treating or trying to prevent osteoporosis have a vitamin D deficiency.

Osteoporosis occurs as bones lose minerals and become weak, brittle, and prone to breaking. As you age, your bones can lose their density, and postmenopausal women lose bone density more quickly than men. Vitamin D's primary role is to ensure that calcium is metabolized in the body and deposited in your bones. If you are deficient in vitamin D, you will not get enough access to calcium no matter how much you ingest. In fact, if you have a vitamin D deficiency, you may only be able to absorb one half to a third of the calcium that you would absorb with healthier vitamin D levels.

Elderly people, especially those living in institutions or who are shut in and have little sun exposure, are at great risk for vitamin D deficiency and, therefore, at risk for osteoporosis and fractures. Osteoporosis is painless and usually a painful fracture is the first sign of the disease.

Earlier, I explained some of the implications for elderly people who have low levels of vitamin D. I also discussed that raising levels has a positive impact on bone health. The studies that I am about to bring up are not prospective ones, but they do show movement toward a connection between vitamin D and issues that are of concern to elderly people (and their families).

It is known that insufficient levels of vitamin D lead to impaired transportation of calcium across the intestines, which causes a decline in circulating calcium. As a result, extra parathyroid hormone is secreted, which is related to the loss and breakdown of bone. After improving vitamin D blood levels from 20 ng/ml to 32 ng/ml, calcium transport in the intestine increases by over 45 percent. Calcium needs vitamin D—without it only 10 to 15 percent of your calcium intake is absorbed. One study showed that maximum bone density was achieved when vitamin D blood levels reached 40 ng/ml in patients.

A Case of Bone Density and Vitamin D Deficiency

Catherine was a 51-year-old executive who came to me because of advanced osteopenia (the precursor to osteoporosis). She had been taking 1,000 milligrams of calcium every day. Her calcium supplement had vitamin D in it, but only 400 units! In addition, she did regular weight-bearing exercises and was taking a low dose of additional vitamin D. However, as is very common with perimenopausal women, her bone density continued to drop little by little every year. Her osteoporosis specialist had told her that if it continued to drop, she would have no choice but to take one of the biphosphonate drugs. Because Catherine was very oriented toward natural health solutions and did not want to take pharmaceutical drugs, she came to me for any insights I might have.

Of course, the first thing I did was measure her vitamin D level. Her vitamin D level was below 10 ng/ml—a severe deficiency. I explained the key role vitamin D plays in maintaining bone health and that without it she could not absorb calcium properly from either her pills or her food. She was shocked that her osteoporosis doctor had not checked her vitamin D level (and so was I). I started Catherine on a therapeutic dose of vitamin D, and over the next months, her blood levels rose to over 50 ng/ml. She continued her calcium supplement and weight-bearing exercises.

The following year, I did a repeat bone density test on Catherine. To our great delight, rather than the persistent progression of slow loss of bone, she had actually gained rather than lost more bone density. It certainly appears in this case, since the vitamin D was the only thing we changed, that this supplementation allowed her better absorption and utilization of her calcium and was a factor in her bone density stabilizing. And at least so far, we have stopped the progressive loss of her bone.

I see many women in their 40s and 50s who have osteopenia. Many of them have been to osteoporosis specialists in the greater Los Angeles area; however, almost none have ever had a vitamin D–level test done and the vast majority are significantly deficient in vitamin D.

Fractures and Falls

In the United States, as the number of elderly people in the population increases, the incidence of fractures related to osteoporosis are expected to increase from more than 2 million in 2005 to more than 3 million in 2025—an increase of 50 percent. The annual medical costs related to this are estimated to grow from $17 billion to approximately $25 billion in 2025. Researchers predict that nearly 47 percent of women over the age of 50 and nearly 22 percent of men over 50 will have an osteoporosis-related fracture.

Of particular concern is the fact that many otherwise healthy people never recover from a hip fracture.

According to statistics gathered by the International Osteoporosis Foundation (IOF), between 20 and 24 percent of people with a hip fracture are likely to die in the first year after the fracture, and their risk of death increases with each year afterward. They continue to have a greater risk of dying for at least five years after the hip fracture.

Those who survive a hip fracture may experience a loss of independence and reduced functioning, with 33 percent requiring nursing home care in the following year. A hip fracture impairs the ability to walk without aid in 40 percent of survivors, and 60 percent continue to require some kind of assistance a year after the hip fracture.

Vertebral fractures are another risk for people over 50 with osteoporosis. These are the types of fractures that can result in deformity in the spine and loss of height. They may also cause back pain and affect daily life and self-image.

Fractures can be debilitating and life threatening to elderly people, and many aging adults are vigilant about getting the recommended dosage of calcium to keep their bones strong. However, the importance of getting enough vitamin D to ensure that calcium can be absorbed so it can get into the bones is underemphasized. The body is unable to build bone mass optimally or maintain strong bones without it.

Several studies have been done with aging populations to determine the effect of vitamin D supplementation on the incidence of fractures. One study indicated that 100 percent of elderly women admitted to the hospital with osteoporotic fractures were deficient in vitamin D, even though half of the women were taking some vitamin D supplementation.

The women in this study who were not taking supplemental vitamin D had severely deficient levels of vitamin D—as low as 11 ng/ml. However, the women who were taking supplements had vitamin D levels of 16 ng/ml, which is not much better. A study published in 2008 reviewed many previous studies that investigated vitamin D and the risk of fracture and reported that levels of more than 30 ng/ml were associated with reduced risk of fractures in elderly people. By comparison, I recommend that all my patients have optimal levels of at least 40 ng/ml all year.

A 1992 study gave 3,270 elderly women a daily supplement of 800 IU of vitamin D and 1,200 mg of calcium for three years. Their risk of hip fracture was reduced by 43 percent, and the risk of nonvertebral fractures was reduced by 32 percent. The results of another study showed a 58 percent decline in nonvertebral fractures when men and women over 65 were supplemented with daily doses of 700 IU of vitamin D and 600 mg of calcium.

Many of my patients who have elderly parents have been concerned about their parents falling (and sustaining fractures) and also cannot help but notice that their parents are seeming to lose strength. Vitamin D levels of less than 20 ng/ml are associated with body sway in the elderly. Researchers have shown that the vitamin D receptors in the muscles perform a series of metabolic actions, which are essential for muscle contraction. When elderly people in a number of studies raised their vitamin D levels to between 26 and 33 ng/ml, their lower-extremity muscle performance appeared to improve.

Studies looked at elderly people living in nursing homes and investigated the effect of vitamin D supplementation on their propensity to fall. One study gave 1,200 IU of daily vitamin D or a placebo to 625 patients whose average age was 83. The group who took the vitamin D had a 27 percent reduced risk of falls. Another study found that 800 IU of daily vitamin D supplementation seemed to reduce falls in the elderly nursing-home patients, but 200 or 400 IU/day did not have any benefit.

A 2007 study measured the vitamin D levels of more than 900 people over 65 years of age and measured their physical performance and their strength using a handgrip. Nearly 29 percent of the women and

14 percent of the men had vitamin D levels below 10 ng/ml—which were considered deficient in the study. Approximately 75 percent of the women and 51 percent of the men had levels below 20 ng/ml, which was considered insufficient in the study (but deficient by current standards). Poor physical performance and strength measures were associated with low levels of vitamin D.

People who were 60 years and older were measured for their walking speed and sit-to-stand times, and those with vitamin D levels above 30 ng/ml were shown to have the best performance.

Osteomalacia

Osteomalacia is also known as adult rickets and is clearly associated with a deficiency in vitamin D. Our bones are constantly remodeling themselves, breaking down, and then rebuilding with new material. In osteoporosis, they do not rebuild as fast as they are broken down, resulting in weak, porous bones. In osteomalacia, when the bones rebuild, they do not harden as they should, and the result is softer bones. Another distinguishing feature is that osteomalacia is associated with deep, chronic muscle and bone pain with tenderness, especially the breastbone (sternum) and the outside of the shin (tibia bone), as well as the forearms.

Some people who have been diagnosed with fibromyalgia, arthritis, and chronic fatigue syndrome are actually just vitamin D deficient and actually have osteomalacia. In one study, 140 out of 150 people in the hospital with persistent muscle and bone pain that was unresponsive to treatment were found to have vitamin D levels averaging 12 ng/ml, which is severely deficient.

Another study noted that 93 percent of people aged 10 to 65 years who entered the emergency room for bone and muscle pain and had been diagnosed with fibromyalgia, depression, and chronic fatigue syndrome were vitamin D deficient.

An article in the *British Medical Journal* described a case where a woman from Pakistan who had been treated for breast cancer continued to suffer from chronic, severe muscle and bone pain for two years following her cancer treatment. She was mistakenly diagnosed with metastatic bone disease and prescribed drugs for it, which did not alleviate the pain. However, a six-week trip to sunny Pakistan served to resolve the condition. Her pain returned in the winter, and it was only then that she was properly diagnosed with osteomalacia and treated for vitamin D deficiency.

Vitamin D and Chronic Pain

The discussion on osteomalacia leads us to the subject of chronic pain and vitamin D deficiency. When I entered the term *chronic pain* into an Internet search engine, there were more than eight million hits. The National Pain Foundation indicates that 25 percent of Americans (75 million) suffer with chronic pain, and that chronic pain issues are the reason for 80 percent of visits to medical doctors. The costs of medical and disability claims and lost productivity associated with this condition are estimated at $70 billion annually.

While I acknowledge that there are many types of chronic pain, I am going to focus on chronic pain that researchers believe to be associated with vitamin D deficiency. In a report prepared for medical professionals, experts indicated that any patient who has unexplained chronic muscle, joint, or bone pain; fibromyalgia; myalgia; or chronic fatigue syndrome should be evaluated for vitamin D deficiency. The authors noted that additional research is still required, but after reviewing 22 existing studies on musculoskeletal pain in more than 3,600 patients, they determined that between 48 and 100 percent of the participants had vitamin D inadequacy.

When the reviewers analyzed these studies of participants who experienced chronic pain, 70 percent had vitamin D levels below 20 ng/ml. Patients with pain had significantly lower vitamin D levels than their counterparts who did not have pain, according to the control studies reviewed. When supplementation of vitamin D was given in the studies, there was significant improvement in pain and muscle strength, and physical performance often improved.

Researchers first suspected a link between musculoskeletal pain and vitamin D deficiency because the pain symptoms appeared to be worse in the winter when vitamin D–making UVB rays were inaccessible. One study that investigated pain showed that every participant aged 10 to 65 years old had symptoms of vitamin D deficiency. One year prior to this study, these patients had been evaluated for chronic pain, but none had been tested for vitamin D deficiency.

A study published in 2003 looked at 360 patients aged 15 to 52 years who experienced lower-back pain for more than six months. Their chronic pain had no known cause. Blood tests were taken measuring vitamin D levels and showed that 83 percent of the patients had "an abnormally low level of vitamin D" before they were given supplements. After supplementation, 95 percent of the patients in the study noted clinical improvement in their lower back pain. The researchers suggested that vitamin D deficiency is linked with lower-back pain, and vitamin D blood levels should be tested in patients who suffer with this condition.

In another study, it was noteworthy that female patients with back pain who weighed more than 110 pounds required twice the vitamin D dose of women who weighed less than 110 pounds in order to achieve the same level of pain relief.

A study looked at the data of patients with knee pain associated with osteoarthritis (OA) who reported having almost daily pain for the month prior to the observation. Researchers found that 48 percent of the patients had vitamin D levels below 20 ng/ml. Those with low levels experienced more pain and disability than those with higher vitamin D levels.

A number of studies indicated that chronic pain was associated with very low levels of vitamin D, with one study reporting that 88 percent of patients reporting chronic pain had less than 10 ng/ml of vitamin D in their blood. At the annual scientific meeting of the American Headache Society in June 2008, a study was presented illustrating that 40 percent of patients with chronic migraines were deficient in vitamin D, with levels below 30 ng/ml. Only 7 percent of migraine sufferers had received adequate vitamin D supplementation. The study also showed that people who had suffered with chronic migraines for the longest time had an increased likelihood of being deficient in vitamin D.

Vitamin D deficiency experts have recommended that physicians consider vitamin D deficiency and its association with osteomalacia as part of the differential diagnosis in all patients with fibromyalgia, chronic musculoskeletal pain, muscle weakness, or fatigue, including chronic fatigue syndrome.

Vitamin D and Autoimmune Diseases

When things are working properly in the body, our immune system protects us from viruses, bacteria, organisms, and, therefore, from illness, disease, and infection. In some people, the immune system becomes faulty and attacks the body it is meant to protect. When this occurs, it is known as autoimmunity.

Everyone has some level of autoimmunity that is not harmful. However, it can lead to autoimmune diseases. According to the American Autoimmune Related Diseases Association, there are about 80 to 100 chronic illnesses known as autoimmune diseases. Such diseases may be present in different muscles, tissues, and nerves, as well as other parts of the body, including the endocrine system (type 1, or insulin-dependent diabetes), the nervous system (multiple sclerosis), or in the joints (rheumatoid arthritis). It is estimated that 23.5 million Americans have autoimmune diseases, and approximately 75 percent of them are women.

The following information will highlight the few autoimmune diseases that have been associated with vitamin D. I will review some of the research conducted on vitamin D and insulin-dependent diabetes and multiple sclerosis, and briefly look at rheumatoid arthritis and inflammatory bowel disease and their possible association with vitamin D.

I want to be very clear that we are in the early days in the study of vitamin D and its possible association with autoimmune diseases. And while I am encouraged by the current research, many more years of prospective studies are required before we can make solid recommendations. I am presenting findings about vitamin D and very specific autoimmune diseases, and I am not generalizing these findings to any of the other autoimmune diseases.

Type 1 Diabetes and Vitamin D

Type 1 diabetes, also known as insulin-dependent diabetes, is a condition that occurs when one's own immune system attacks the pancreas and destroys the islet cells that produce insulin. This form of diabetes usually occurs in childhood or adolescence but may hit at any age. Experts do not know what causes type

1 diabetes, but the Juvenile Diabetes Research Foundation has funded research looking into whether or not vitamin D deficiency is a risk factor.

Currently there is not a known cure for type 1 diabetes, and it appears that its prevalence is on the rise. By the time a diagnosis is made, it is estimated that 80 percent of the insulin-producing cells have already been destroyed. A 2008 study indicated that the worldwide incidence of insulin-dependent diabetes is increasing by 3 percent annually, and by 2010, rates of this disease could be 40 percent higher than they were in 2000.

Vitamin D expert Dr. John Cannell points out that the rise of insulin-dependent diabetes reached epidemic levels after warnings about sun avoidance became pervasive. Furthermore, it is more likely to be diagnosed in the fall and winter when there is minimal sun exposure, and it is less likely to be diagnosed in summer. Epidemiological studies have indicated that the incidence of type 1 diabetes is more prevalent in higher latitudes. There is shocking evidence when you compare the incidence of diabetes in Finland and Venezuela. Children in Finland are nearly 400 times more likely to have insulin-dependent diabetes than children in Venezuela. Northern Finland sits at 67 degrees latitude (far from the equator), and Venezuela is at 6 degrees latitude.

Until 1964, the Finnish government's recommendation of vitamin D for children in Finland was up to 5,000 IU/day at which time it was reduced to 2,000 IU/day, apparently for safety reasons rather than observed toxicity. In 1975, the level was reduced to 1,000 IU/day; and finally, in 1992, the recommendation for infants was lowered to 400 IU/day.

In 1966, before the drastic reductions in Finland's recommendations for vitamin D, a study was launched of more than 10,000 pregnant mothers. Medical information about their infants was also charted, including their intake of vitamin D during their first year of life. Thirty years later, between 1997 and 1998, researchers led by Elina Hyppönen retrospectively reviewed the medical information and published the results. The children who had been among the recipients of the 2,000 IU/day recommended dose for infants had an approximate 80 percent reduced risk of developing juvenile diabetes. Researchers compared diabetes-incidence rates from the time children received 2,000 IU/day to incidence rates after the daily recommendation had been dropped to 400 IU/day and found a fivefold increase in the incidence of insulin-dependent diabetes.

Observational studies indicate that children may have a higher risk of developing insulin-dependent diabetes if their mothers had low intakes of vitamin D during pregnancy. Children whose mothers had taken either vitamin D supplementation or cod-liver oil (a source of vitamin D) during pregnancy were less likely to develop insulin-dependent diabetes than those whose mothers did not take vitamin D supplementation.

In an audio interview discussing his recent journal article on vitamin D and juvenile diabetes, Dr. Cedric Garland suggested that vitamin D may interact with certain types of white blood cells and enable them to act as "peacemakers" in the tissues of the pancreas. If a child has sufficient levels of vitamin D, the peacemaker cells are likely to be more abundant and will, therefore, stop the immune system from attacking the cells that produce insulin in the pancreas. If there is not enough vitamin D, which can be the case in northern latitudes, there may not be enough peacemaker cells to fight off an attack on the insulin-making cells of the pancreas.

According to Dr. Garland: "We are in a position in our modern technological society, to head off this disease and to prevent it safely under the care of a physician, and even to prevent it without the care of a physician, if everything is done with great prudence. It seems a great shame to hold back, based on the studies we have acquired."

At the time of this writing, prospective randomized-control studies have not been conducted on vitamin D and insulin-dependent diabetes; therefore, we can only say that vitamin D deficiency in an infant appears to be strongly associated with an increased risk for type 1 diabetes. However, so far, researchers who are investigating the connection between vitamin D and type 1 diabetes have not found any other reason to explain the skyrocketing incidence of this disease in children. The evidence is all pointing to vitamin D deficiency as a significant predisposing factor, and I agree that it is important to take these studies to heart and do our best as physicians to prevent the risk to children from this lifelong condition.

About Type 2 Diabetes

While type 2 diabetes is not an autoimmune disease, it bears mentioning here. Type 2 diabetes is typically linked with an unhealthy lifestyle and obesity, and used to occur primarily in adults in later life. With the current epidemic in childhood obesity, however, it is now also being diagnosed in children. A review study published in 2007 indicated that there may be evidence connecting type 2 diabetes mellitus with vitamin D levels and calcium. Observational studies that were reviewed suggest that vitamin D and calcium may improve insulin resistance and systemic inflammation but are unclear about the mechanisms involved.

An Australian study found that avoiding the sun could be increasing people's risk for type 2 diabetes. Lower levels of vitamin D in the blood could be associated with higher blood-glucose levels.

In another study, 51 patients with type 2 diabetes and neuropathic nerve pain characterized by burning, tingling, throbbing, and numbness were all found to be severely vitamin D deficient with blood levels averaging below 18 ng/ml. After three months of daily doses of 2,000 IU of vitamin D, pain scores were cut almost in half. The authors of the study suggested that vitamin D could be considered a side-effect free analgesic for patients with type 2 diabetic neuropathic pain, as well as a preventive treatment for osteoporosis to which people with diabetes are prone.

And in yet another study, the risk for developing type 2 diabetes was lowered by 33 percent with 800 IU of vitamin D and 1,200 mg of calcium taken daily. Taking half of the these doses did not have an impact on lowering risk.

Multiple Sclerosis

Multiple sclerosis (MS) is a degenerative autoimmune disease that affects the central nervous system, specifically the myelin, which protects the brain and the spinal cord. According to the Multiple Sclerosis Association of America, an estimated 400,000 people in the United States have MS. Incidence is correlated with latitude, with North America, Europe, and southern Australia having higher rates than people in Asia, which is closer to the equator. On average, MS affects three times more women than men.

Growing up and living below 35 degrees of latitude for the first ten years of life reduces a person's chance of getting MS by about 50 percent. Several studies have verified that the lower the blood levels of vitamin D in youth, the more increased the risk of developing MS in adulthood. Children in Tasmania who had the highest exposure to UVB rays, which are responsible for making vitamin D, had an almost 70 percent reduced risk of developing multiple sclerosis compared to children who had sun exposure of less than one hour daily.

One study showed that white men and women decreased their risk of developing multiple sclerosis by 41 percent for every increase of 20 ng/ml in their vitamin D blood levels above 24 ng/ml. In another study, women who took 400 IU/day of vitamin D were shown to reduce their risk of developing MS by 42 percent.

One report discusses 12 patients with MS in the active phase who were given increasing doses of vitamin D over 28 weeks. The doses began at 4,000 IU daily and increased to 40,000 IU daily. Their blood vitamin D levels increased from 31 ng/ml to 154 ng/ml on average, and the patients remained without toxic side effects of excess vitamin D. After 28 weeks, the number of MS lesions had decreased to an average of 0.83 from 1.75. Obviously, these high dosage treatments require close physician supervision.

Harvard researchers found that the subjects who had at least 40 ng/ml of vitamin D in their blood at 20 years of age had a greatly reduced risk of MS. Sufficient levels of vitamin D in pregnant women and their infants is also connected to a significantly reduced risk of the infant developing multiple sclerosis later in life.

Vitamin D was shown to be a possible treatment for MS symptoms, as studies indicated that people with MS have more lesions in the winter than the summer, which was linked to the availability of UVB access and vitamin D synthesis.

Other Autoimmune Diseases

Recent findings show that there may be an association between other autoimmune diseases, including rheumatoid arthritis and inflammatory bowel disease, and vitamin D deficiency. However, these studies are in their infancy.

Vitamin D and Mental Health

As with most tissues in the body, there are vitamin D receptors in the brain. Low levels of vitamin D have been linked to an increased risk for depression and schizophrenia, which could increase the importance of having sufficient levels of vitamin D available to a growing fetus and to infants.

In one animal study, severe vitamin D deficiency in pregnant animals was linked to brain abnormality in their offspring. Abnormal apoptosis and brain-cell proliferation were observed as well as learning and memory problems. In another animal study, the brain abnormalities observed in rat pups whose mothers were severely deficient in vitamin D had similarities to those abnormalities observed in the brains of human children with autism.

As a note about autism and its links to vitamin D, Dr. John Cannell has been developing a theory that there is a relationship between vitamin D deficiency and the rising incidence of autism in children. This is just a theory, however, and is untested by researchers. Such studies are just getting under way, and more will be required before we can make any conclusions.

Researchers are also looking into a possible connection between vitamin D deficiency and schizophrenia.

In fact, an Australian study was announced where researchers will retrospectively look at the blood tests that were taken from newborns who developed schizophrenia as young adults. The researchers will measure vitamin D levels to determine whether there is any connection between vitamin D and schizophrenia in humans.

Cognitive Impairment in the Aged

In a study of memory and aging, participants with Alzheimer's disease were compared with people who did not have the disease. Several tests of cognitive function were conducted as well as a physical performance test. Vitamin D blood levels were also measured with the average at approximately 18 ng/ml. More than half of the participants had vitamin D levels below 20 ng/ml. Those with a vitamin D deficiency had worse scores in cognitive performance, and their deficiency was associated with an active mood disorder. Another study found that 4,000 IU/day of vitamin D improved the mood of elderly patients.

Vitamin D and Seasonal Affective Disorder

Seasonal Affective Disorder (SAD) is a form of depression that occurs seasonally in the winter months and is associated with low levels of sunlight. People often refer to the "winter blues" to describe the phenomenon of SAD. According to Mental Health America, three out of four people who have SAD are women. SAD is less prevalent the closer you live to the equator, and rare within 30 degrees latitude of the equator.

SAD is often misdiagnosed as severe depression or bipolar disorder, as well as illnesses such as hypothyroidism, hypoglycemia, mononucleosis, and other viral infections. Symptoms associated with SAD are far reaching and include depression, anxiety, sexual problems, overeating, and oversleeping. The disorder is typically treated with light therapy or antidepressants.

SAD is also linked to the production of melatonin, which is produced in the dark by the pineal gland. More melatonin is produced at times of the year when the days are shorter. Being exposed to sunlight suppresses melatonin and may be partly responsible for the good feelings that being in the sun can create. In addition, sun exposure has been found to stimulate dopamine, serotonin, and beta-endorphins, which may also stimulate mood.

When people with SAD are exposed to the UVB light from tanning beds, their vitamin D levels increased and the SAD symptoms improved.

A Case of Stress and Fatigue Alleviated by Vitamin D

I have been discussing serious diseases and illnesses and their relationship to vitamin D. And while I have not seen this in any study, I have observed that the quality of life and well-being of many of my patients has also improved as their vitamin D levels are optimized.

Most of my patients have busy lives, and although they may be otherwise healthy, they do experience high levels of fatigue from job pressures and the general stress of life. John was such a patient. He runs a big corporation in Los Angeles. His physical exam and regular blood tests were normal, but his vitamin D level came back at 15 ng/ml. We discussed this, and I told John that I could give him herbs to help with fatigue, but I suggested that we try correcting his vitamin D level first and see how he felt.

Two weeks later, John returned to go over some other test results. He said, "Doc, I can't believe this. After two weeks of the high-dose vitamin D, my energy has remarkably improved. I have never seen anything like it!"

I, too, had never seen anything so dramatic as just taking the right dose of vitamin D to improve a patient's energy levels. It would be another two months before John's blood level was totally corrected, but his level had been so low that just two weeks of the high dose treatment had produced a dramatic improvement in his fatigue. Subsequent herbs were not required.

It has been quite a while since John's vitamin D level were optimized, but he still tells all his friends about the benefits of vitamin D!

Vitamin D and Skin Conditions

Psoriasis is a skin condition characterized by thick, raised patches of red, itchy skin with scaly patches called plaques. An old remedy for psoriasis was sun exposure. Dr. Michael Holick developed a pharmaceutical cream containing activated vitamin D to use as an ointment for people with this condition. This is a drug and is available by prescription from your doctor.

While writing this book, I received a testimonial from the daughter of my patient Florence with a rare skin condition called Grover's disease. Florence gave me permission to include the following letter written by her daughter:

Florence is an 80-year-old patient of Dr. Khalsa. For the past ten years, she has suffered from severe itching. When it first began, she went to two different dermatologists and was diagnosed with "Grover's disease." She was prescribed various antihistamines, and even antidepressants. Nothing worked. The itching got worse and worse to the point where she had trouble sleeping. She thought it might be an allergy to her bed, so she purchased a new one. She got no relief. She changed her air conditioning in the house and got a whole new system with very expensive filters. That didn't work. She moved out of her house into a hotel to see if something else at home was the source, but that didn't help either. She got rid of her two dogs whom she adored, thinking that she must be allergic to them. The itching persisted. In some seasons, it was worse than others.

Four years ago (2004), she and her husband moved into a condo and left their house, partly because her husband was aging and needed a home that was more accommodating to his needs—and partly due to my mom's itching. She thought maybe their house was unhealthy for her. Recently, Dr. Khalsa tested her vitamin D level. It was extremely low. He put her on a course of vitamin D supplements and within two days of treatment, she was markedly better. Her vitamin D is now at normal levels, and her itching is 98 percent better. She still gets occasional itching, but it's miraculously better. God bless Dr. Khalsa!

Vitamin D and Teeth

Preliminary investigations indicate that there may be a relationship between maternal vitamin D levels during pregnancy and tooth decay in children at about 16 months of age. Another study indicated that low levels of vitamin D could be associated with periodontal disease.

Asthma in Children

A report about a study of children with asthma was released in July 2008. Children had been selected to participate in a drug trial testing two inhaled asthma medications. Although the intention of the experiment was not to examine the relationship between vitamin D and asthma, researchers tested the vitamin D levels of children before they were randomly placed in groups for the drug trial. Those with levels below 30 ng/ml were considered to be vitamin D deficient, and it was noted that 30 percent of the children had levels below 30 ng/ml.

The study found that during the drug trial, 24 percent of the children who had insufficient vitamin D levels experienced a severe asthma reaction requiring hospitalization or an emergency-room visit, whereas only 18 percent of the children with sufficient levels had a severe asthma reaction.

When the researchers adjusted for other factors, they found that children with insufficient levels of vitamin D had about a 70 percent increased risk of having severe asthma reactions compared to the children with sufficient levels. Sufficient levels of vitamin D may have also been linked to the number of days the children were free of asthma symptoms.

Vitamin D and Influenza

Until recently, the seasonal increase of influenza cases, prevalent in the Northern Hemisphere between December and March, has stumped conventional medicine. Doctors postulated that it was primarily due to the extremely cold weather and the tendency for people to get less fresh air. Now researchers believe that vitamin D's ability to boost the immune system may explain the phenomenon.

This connection was first made in 1992 by physician and researcher R. Edgar Hope-Simpson, M.D. After studying widespread flu epidemics of the past, Dr. Hope-

Simpson proposed that a "seasonal stimulus" was the culprit. He suggested that this "seasonal stimulus" had to do with how much sunshine people got in winter, and that the lack of sunshine increased their likelihood of contracting influenza. Although he recognized that the virus was spread through contact, he believed that the "seasonal stimulus" was actually the real root cause. This link explains why influenza breakouts occurred simultaneously in disparate areas throughout history—something that has always stumped scientists.

At the time Dr. Hope-Simpson made his observations, researchers had yet to find the link between vitamin D and human immunity. Since then research has shown that vitamin D has a positive effect on the immune system by giving a boost to the macrophages (bacteria-killing white blood cells). Experts also believe that vitamin D enhances the body's natural antibiotic molecules that exist in the lining of the respiratory tract, among other places. Similarly, vitamin D has been shown to reduce the frequency of respiratory infections in children.

Dr. John Cannell wrote about his experience in April 2005 in the psychiatric hospital where he works. A flu epidemic broke out in the hospital, requiring many wards to be quarantined. He noticed that none of the patients on his ward had contracted the flu despite the fact that they had contact with other patients who were ill before the quarantine was implemented. Dr. Cannell's patients were similar to all of the other patients in the hospital and had similar medications and backgrounds.

However, one thing was different. His patients had all been taking 2,000 IU of vitamin D, on his prescription, for several months before the flu epidemic. Now this is just an observation, and certainly not science, but one cannot help but wonder whether vitamin D had an impact on the fact that not a single patient of his fell ill.

Dr. Cannell launched his own investigation and co-wrote an article with a team of vitamin D experts to discuss their theories about the connection between vitamin D and influenza. They hypothesized that influenza was a "symptom" of vitamin D deficiency and could be responsible for the predictable, seasonal nature of the illness.

I want to reiterate that this is just a theory, and while it will likely launch further studies into the links between vitamin D, the flu, and the common cold, no one is in a position to make any final conclusions. However, if there is a possibility that 2,000 IU/day of vitamin D could help combat winter colds and flu, I am all for taking it!

A Case of Recurrent Flu

A 50-year-old secretary came to me in October saying that she wanted to "boost her immune system" for the upcoming flu season. She said that she usually comes down with the flu two or three times every year, and even getting the flu shot did not seem to prevent it.

Of course, I measured her vitamin D level, and it was 11 ng/ml—very low! I immediately started her on a corrective dose of vitamin D and had her repeat the test in January. Indeed, her levels had gotten up to 50 ng/ml.

In May of the next year, she sent me a note that said: "The vitamin D you gave me, Dr. Khalsa, is amazing! This is the first year in ten years that I haven't gotten the flu once. Thank you so much for discovering this deficiency. I'm telling all of my friends about it."

A Case of Sinusitis

Michael, a 25-year-old man, came to me because he had endured eight sinus infections in the previous 12 months for a total of 80 days of antibiotics in the last year. He, too, was seeking "immune support." Michael's vitamin D level probably was extraordinarily low at 9 ng/ml because he has an indoor job and also has fair skin.

I immediately started him on a corrective dose of vitamin D. In addition, he began a series of acupuncture and herbal treatments as well as dietary changes. I am very happy to report that in the seven months since he first came to see me, he has only had one sinus infection with this protocol.

Michael has educated himself about vitamin D by reading articles that I have directed him to, in addition to ones published in the *New York Times* and *Wall Street Journal*. During his last visit to my office, he remarked, "Dr. Khalsa, why didn't my sinus doctor measure my vitamin D level?"

Michael is now encouraging all his friends to take at least a basic supportive dose of vitamin D.

◻◼◻

Dr. Cannell and his research team summarized their findings (in the journal *Expert Opinion Pharmacotherapy*) on vitamin D levels and their impact on illnesses and disease. The following chart shows a summary of their review of the medical literature and the associated benefits for disease prevention at different vitamin D blood levels.

Ideal Vitamin D (25D) Levels Related to Health Issues	
Issue	Vitamin D Levels
Rickets and Osteomalacia	15 ng/ml
Supress parathyroid hormone levels	20–30 ng/ml
Optimize intestinal calcium absorption	34 ng/ml
Improve neuromuscular performance in elderly	38 ng/ml
Reduction of incidence of internal cancer	38 ng/ml
50 percent lower risk of colon cancer	33 ng/ml
50 percent reduction in breast-cancer incidence	52 ng/ml

▫▪▫

I have given you a lot of information and facts on illnesses, diseases, and vitamin D deficiency. Remember that the good news is that vitamin D deficiency is relatively easy to correct. It may take a few months, but I have never had a patient who did not respond with improved vitamin D blood levels. In the following chapter, I will talk about diagnosing a deficiency and share the recommendations that I give my own patients to correct their vitamin D levels.

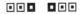

Chapter Five

MEASURING VITAMIN D DEFICIENCY AND OPTIMIZING VITAMIN D LEVELS

By this point in the book, I hope that you—like me and so many of the vitamin D researchers I have introduced—understand why it is so important to normalize and even optimize your own vitamin D level. You now know that diagnosing and treating a vitamin D deficiency in yourself and in your loved ones could provide many great health benefits.

Diagnosing a Vitamin D Deficiency

Whether you are a healthy person who wants to stay that way or someone who has one of the vitamin D–associated illnesses or diseases, I hope that you will want to evaluate, and if necessary, treat your own vitamin D deficiency.

Looking in the mirror and seeing that you have fair skin or a suntan might give you some idea on the status of your vitamin D level. However, this could be very misleading and will only be a guess. Fair-skinned people who get 50 percent of their full-body minimal erythemal dose (MED) several times a week will probably have a normal vitamin D level, but they will not at all appear sunburned or suntanned.

Similarly, people who are naturally more dark skinned or have a suntan may assume that they are getting plenty of vitamin D, but they may in fact be deficient. Indeed, as I mentioned earlier, darker-skinned individuals have more melanin in their skin, which serves as a natural sunblock. The only real way to find out if you are deficient in vitamin D is with a blood test of 25-hydroxyvitamin D.

For decades, physicians in medical schools have been taught to draw a 1,25-dihydroxyvitamin D level as the way to test for vitamin D in the body. But all of the medical literature over the last ten years now indicates that this particular test does not give an accurate picture of the vitamin D stores in your body; rather, it is merely a reflection of the kidney's function.

The consensus of all vitamin D research is that the only reliable blood test to evaluate vitamin D is the 25-hydroxyvitamin D (25D) test. The blood levels in the studies that I have cited throughout this book have always used this test.

In the best scenario, you would be able to go to your physician and request a blood test. If your doctor is not willing to do the blood test, then perhaps you could ask for a lab requisition so that you may go to a lab yourself and have the test done. At the time of printing, a very popular national laboratory charges approximately $200 for this service.

However, with the direction that managed care is taking us in our current society, many patients are increasingly realizing the importance and need for self-care. Today, a woman can do a home pregnancy test to see if she is pregnant without consulting her obstetrician. Similarly, many patients with high blood pressure can buy an inexpensive device to check their own blood pressure at home. For many years, diabetics have monitored their own blood sugar with finger-stick home tests. In each of these cases, patients are able to gather a lot of information by themselves. Many individuals are managing their own medical issues and only call on their physician if they need help or guidance.

Some patients may have a doctor who is not knowledgeable about vitamin D and who will not "allow" them to get a vitamin D blood test. Similarly, many people may not want to go to a physician and pay for an office visit just to get a blood test.

In keeping with the trend for patient self-care and home testing, a new home self-test kit for checking your vitamin D level has been developed. It is known as a "blood spot" home test. It does not give you an immediate answer in the way that a pregnancy test or a blood-sugar test does. Rather, with this test, you prick your own finger (with a small, sterile lancet provided by the lab), and you put several drops of your blood on special blotter paper that is provided. Once it dries, you simply send it to the laboratory. Within approximately two weeks, the results of your 25D test result will come to you by mail.

At this point, you can either bring the test results to your physician to review and decide on treatment, if any, or you may decide to begin treatment yourself because vitamin D is inexpensive and easily available over the counter.

It is my hope that with this self-test kit, we can bring about worldwide normalization of everyone's vitamin D level. So, what would happen if we implemented treatment to normalize the entire population's vitamin D level? As I have mentioned, the well-respected vitamin D researcher Robert Heaney, M.D., has stated that until we normalize everybody's vitamin D status, we will not really know what the true incidence of disease could be in North America. I would like to expand this notion to include the health of the entire world!

Whether you are a resident of Canada or Scandinavia and only spend time in the sun during the summer months, or a pregnant woman in the Middle East or India whose tradition requires you to wear clothing that fully covers the body, imagine what it would be like if the entire world's population had normal vitamin D levels!

Measuring Vitamin D Levels

There are several technologies used to measure 25D. For a long time, simple radioimmunoassay (RIA) was the standard way to measure 25D. However, in the last couple of years, two even more accurate technologies have been developed. The first is called liquid chromatography-tandem mass spectrometry (LC-MS/MS), and the second is the DiaSorin Liaison test. Both of these technologies, when run carefully by a laboratory, provide very accurate results for vitamin D levels. The national laboratory I briefly mentioned as well as the at-home test kit I described use these new technologies.

A third-party organization called the Vitamin D External Quality Assessment Scheme (DEQAS) has also been formed. The overall goal of DEQAS is to ensure the analytical reliability of 25-hydroxyvitamin D assays.

They issue performance-proficiency certificates to laboratories for their vitamin D testing. Labs that wish to obtain this certification are sent serum samples to test at regular intervals, and then they return their results to DEQAS. The labs that have obtained accurate results for the specimens sent to them are then certified by the organization. I am happy to report that the lab I work with and the home-test blood-spot lab have both obtained their performance-proficiency certificates from DEQAS.

If you do a blood test with your physician, be sure to confirm that the lab your doctor's office uses has been DEQAS certified. This will ensure that the results on which you are basing your treatment will be accurate.

When to Test Your Vitamin D Level

If you have never had a 25D blood test and you want to begin monitoring your vitamin D level, then any time of the year is a great time to do so. This will give you a baseline, a starting point from which to launch your journey toward vitamin D sufficiency or optimization. Do not be surprised if your vitamin D level is very low! Remember that my initial level was only 11 ng/ml! After taking a supplement for a while, you can then remeasure your blood and see how you are progressing. After making a positive change in your vitamin D level, you can then create a seasonal schedule of testing, which I will discuss.

If you are getting a lot of sunshine in the summer in the United States and allowing yourself some time in the sun without sunblock, your vitamin D level may well be normal. A good time to check your level would be in the late fall or approximately October or November, depending on where you live. Winter is coming, and you will want to make sure that your vitamin D stores are adequate.

If your latitude is north of the 35th parallel, you enter your "vitamin D winter" by November. At this time of year, even if you sit outside in the sun, you will not get any vitamin D. I recommend that my patients take at least 2,000 IU of vitamin D every day throughout the entire winter starting in November.

I would also recommend another vitamin D blood test—especially if you live in the northern latitudes—in March at the end of winter. This is kind of your report card to see how you did during the winter season.

If your levels have dropped, you can begin to correct them. If your levels were maintained over the winter and you are going to be out in the sun in the spring and summer, you can most likely stop your supplementary oral vitamin D.

In summary, I recommend that you measure your vitamin D in the fall and spring unless you are new to testing your level. In that case, test yourself immediately, and then take the necessary steps to normalize your level if it is low.

What Is a Normal Vitamin D Level?

If you go to a lab in the United States, and get a vitamin D blood test, the lower end of the normal (as opposed to optimal) range will come back as being between 20 and 30 ng/ml. It is well agreed by all vitamin D researchers—even by the most conservative ones—that below 20 ng/ml is deficient. Below 10 ng/ml is considered severely deficient and associated with rickets and osteomalacia.

However, with all of the information you have been given in this book, which comes from the last ten years of medical literature, the majority of vitamin D researchers worldwide are recommending that the low end of the normal range be set at 30 ng/ml or higher. This comes from many studies showing that levels much higher than 20 ng/ml are required to activate not only the calcium mechanisms that vitamin D affects, but also all of the other autocrine functions of vitamin D.

Autocrine means that a cell is able to make its own chemical messengers (in this case, activated vitamin D) that bind to receptors inside the same cell and lead to changes in the cell's biochemical functioning. This is in contrast to endocrine, where one organ will secrete a molecule (such as a hormone) that has an effect on another distant organ. In all, it is recognized that more than 26 different tissues, including all the organs I have discussed in earlier chapters, can be affected by vitamin D.

Currently, there is not a consensus among researchers on what the minimum blood level of vitamin D should be. Some say 20 ng/ml, some say 30 ng/ml, and others maintain that 40 ng/ml is ideal. Despite this variation, all of the current research indicates that in order to fully activate the autocrine functions, a blood level of at least 40 ng/ml is required.

There is data that supports the recommendation for maintaining even higher levels than 40 ng/ml, including a study I mentioned earlier by Dr. Cedric Garland and others, which estimated that there could be a 50 percent reduction in the incidence of breast cancer if women kept their vitamin D level over 52 ng/ml. Of course, more prospective randomized-controlled trials must be done to confirm this information.

However, I want to make it clear that the majority of the medical literature does not recommend such high levels at this time. Levels of 30 to 40 ng/ml are considered by most researchers to be where the levels should be kept.

The integrative-medicine doctors whom I work with have a different opinion. They believe that although 30 ng/ml is considered "normal" today, an even higher level—one that optimizes vitamin D—should be strived for. The current consensus among these integrative-medicine doctors, including integrative oncologists, is that blood levels should be over 40 ng/ml (some are even saying 50 ng/ml) and as high as 80 ng/ml in order to optimize the functions that vitamin D produces in the body. Supporting this is a study by Dr. Bruce Hollis and others, who found that the vitamin D pathways in 50 percent of people did not get totally "saturated" until the blood level was at least 40 ng/ml.

I realize that most conservative vitamin D researchers who say that anything greater than 20 ng/ml is normal will of course utterly reject the suggestion that levels should be kept over 50 ng/ml. But I do not agree with them! I suspect that this is where the numbers will be going.

I encourage the skeptics to remember that Mother Nature provides these levels to people whose job or lifestyle exposes them to unblocked sun on a regular basis. Studies show that vitamin D levels over 50 ng/ml are not uncommon in outdoor workers. In fact, in one study, patients in a sun-rich environment had levels over 70 ng/ml.

I further support this recommendation because overdose of vitamin D is not seen until blood levels are greater than 100 ng/ml, and true toxicity does not develop until blood levels are over 150 ng/ml. Therefore, the recommendation of 40–70 ng/ml is not harmful or outlandish. At worst, it may just be unnecessary.

As this book is going to press, a groundbreaking editorial commentary written by John Cannell, M.D., Edward Giovannucci, M.D., and 15 other leading vitamin D researchers was just published. In this article they recommend that all children be given sufficient vitamin D to maintain their 25D levels above 50 ng/ml. Furthermore, it was their stated opinion that children with chronic illnesses such as diabetes, autism, or frequent recurrent infections be given sufficient vitamin D to maintain their levels at 65 ng/ml.

I know that this will also be controversial in the medical community. However, I do suspect in the next relatively short period of time that vitamin D levels greater than 50 ng/ml will become accepted as the optimal level for everyone of all ages.

Please check the Website associated with this book (**www.VitaminDRevolution.com**) for updates. You can also register for e-mail updates from me on the latest vitamin D recommendations. New information on this discussion will be posted on my blog, which supports this book.

What Blood Level Do I Strive for in My Patients?

In my own medical practice, I work to ensure that all of my patients have a 25-hydroxy D (25D) level over 40 ng/ml. However, in my patients who have a vitamin D–connected disease such as osteoporosis or cancer, I endeavor to get their levels over 50 ng/ml. I say *endeavor* because as I have mentioned, it is easy to get low levels above 30 ng/ml, but taking the same amount of oral vitamin D does not equally continue to raise levels above 30 at the same rate. In my practice, when I keep patients at high blood levels, they are usually on high doses of vitamin D—up to 4,000 IU per day—and I test their blood every three months to ensure their blood levels stay in the 50 to 70 ng/ml range.

It seems like every week, new information comes out about vitamin D. The optimal blood level is regularly discussed in current medical literature. I plan to include the most cutting-edge data on my Website, and I sincerely expect that on my blog, there will be an active dialogue about these "normal ranges" over the months and years ahead. I look forward to receiving *your* comments as a reader of this book.

Correcting Vitamin D Deficiency

Naturally, an ideal way to correct your vitamin D deficiency would be to get the exact amount of sun needed to raise your level. In his book *The UV Advantage,* Michael Holick, M.D., Ph.D., has outlined a very systematic way—based on your skin type, latitude, season of the year, and time of day—for you to expose yourself to the sun in order to get an optimal amount of vitamin D without allowing yourself to burn. There are also Websites that provide similar information.

The problem with promoting sun exposure is that dermatologists in the American Academy of Dermatology advise all of us to avoid unprotected sun exposure! In light of that, I would be wrong to recommend a lot of sun exposure to my patients even though I feel that incorporating low-dose exposure can be good for our health.

If you choose to use sun exposure to increase your vitamin D level, please do note that it requires very few minutes of sunshine for most people to get a significant rise in their blood levels. As I noted earlier, a mere 15 minutes of summer midday sun or artificial UVB radiation (as in tanning salons) on both sides of the body can provide you with as much as 10,000 to 15,000 IU of vitamin D. Your level of exposure, however, must be calculated with the above variables in mind. People choosing this approach should understand that regular ultraviolet exposure causes aging in the skin and increases the risk of skin cancers.

All of this information also applies to the sun you get at tanning parlors, and the same principle of attaining 25 to 50 percent of your MED (minimal erythemal dose) should be applied if you do visit a tanning salon, as long as you accept the risks discussed.

Food and Vitamin D

Food is not really a good source of vitamin D. As I have explained, vitamin D occurs naturally in a limited number of foods, including selected fatty-fish species (such as salmon, herring, and sardines), fish-liver oil, and sun-dried shiitake mushrooms. Some foods such as milk and certain brands of orange juice are fortified with up to 100 IU of D_3 per eight ounces. There is much advocacy in the medical literature to increase the quantity of vitamin D in fortified foods, which may make these foods a better source of vitamin D in the future.

However, at the current fortification level of 100 IU per eight ounces of milk, a person would have to drink ten glasses of milk per day to get 1,000 IU of vitamin D.

The amounts of vitamin D in food are not high enough to make a significant impact on your vitamin D level. If you are interested in optimizing your vitamin D level, it is unlikely that you will be able to do so with food, no matter how many vitamin D–rich items you eat. Please refer to the chart in Chapter 2 to review the low levels of vitamin D in various food.

Treating Vitamin D Deficiency in My Patients

In my opinion, the best treatment for vitamin D deficiency is vitamin D_3 supplements. As stated earlier in the book, vitamin D_2 (called ergocalciferol) pills are also available. However, vitamin D_2 is considered to be weaker than vitamin D_3. Vitamin D_2 is not naturally found in the human body and is estimated to be about half as effective as D_3 in raising blood levels. For these reasons I exclusively used D_3 in my practice. Of course, I follow blood levels with regularity.

When I prescribe someone 2,000 IU of vitamin D, it sounds like a very large quantity, but in fact, it is only 50 micrograms (1 microgram equals 40 IU). (One thousand micrograms is equal to one milligram.) Compare a dose of 50 micrograms with a typical aspirin, which contains 320 milligrams. Indeed, when you realize this, you can see that I am not talking about massive quantities of vitamin D, in spite of the fact that the international unit (IU) numbers appear to be very large.

The amount of vitamin D needed by a given patient varies by body weight and specifically body fat, as well as the patient's age. In addition, unlike sun exposure, with oral treatment of vitamin D deficiency, it is possible, although very unlikely, to become toxic.

Overweight individuals will require a higher maintenance dose of vitamin D to maintain their blood levels, and people who are obese often need as much as twice the oral dose of vitamin D to normalize and maintain their levels.

Because aging weakens the ability of the skin to make vitamin D, an older person may need a higher dose of vitamin D than a younger person, assuming that both are getting some sun exposure. And darker-skinned people will usually require a higher regular dose of vitamin D than fair-skinned individuals, assuming both are getting some sun.

Vitamin D_3 pills are readily available in the United States in health-food stores and via the Internet. One problem, however, is that the amount of vitamin D in each capsule as labeled on the bottle may not be accurate unless independent certificates of analysis are done by the releasing vitamin company. In one study, the amount of vitamin D in various pill samples was actually only 83 percent of what was stated on the label.

If a typical person takes 1,000 IU of vitamin D per day, it will usually result in a 10 ng/ml elevation of their serum vitamin D level after it has been taken for three to four months. For example, patients with an initial blood level of 10 ng/ml would generally require at least 2,000 IU/day for several months to get their level up to 30 ng/ml, which is the minimum sufficient level. If patients starting with a level of 10 ng/ml wanted to achieve a level of 40 ng/ml, they would need approximately 3,000 IU a day for three to four months to achieve that level. All of this is without UVB skin exposure.

All of this information is relevant when I am correcting my patients' vitamin D levels. However, because we have easy availability of blood tests, I am able to monitor their starting levels and progress as I treat them. Because I am not your physician and, of course, in no way can take responsibility for your health care, I encourage you to speak with a health-care provider who is knowledgeable about correcting your vitamin D level.

What I would like to do here, however, is demonstrate the process I go through in correcting my patients' vitamin D levels.

How I Correct My Patients' Vitamin D Levels

As I have explained, I try to get my patients' vitamin D levels over 40 ng/ml because I, along with many of my integrative-medicine colleagues, feel that this is the optimal level. When you have your blood tested using 25-hydroxyvitamin D (25D), your results will appear as a number, most likely between 10 and 50 ng/ml (nanograms per milliliter).

The following are my recommendations to my patients. I am sharing this information with you so that you can use it as a reference as you and your health-care provider work toward correcting your own vitamin D level. These are guidelines I set out for my patients and are not to be interpreted as recommendations to you personally.

1. If my patients' blood test shows their 25D level to be below 20 ng/ml: This is obviously extremely low. I treat these patients in the way that Dr. Michael Holick has described in his writings and lectures. Specifically, I will prescribe 50,000 IU of vitamin D *per week* for eight weeks. In my office, I will do this by giving patients one prescription-strength vitamin D_3 pill containing 50,000 units per week.

When my patients tell their friends or any other doctor they may know that I am giving them 50,000 IU a week, their eyes bug out! Those who are not familiar with the current medical literature fear that such a large dose will be toxic. In fact, it actually averages out to less than 8,000 IU per day, which will never make an otherwise healthy person with vitamin D deficiency toxic over eight weeks.

Because vitamin D is fat soluble and stored in the body—and specifically 25-hydroxyvitamin D has a half-life of approximately two weeks in the body—this once-a-week dose is very effective but not always easy for my patients to remember.

However, an equally good way to take 50,000 units a week would be to take 5,000 IU of vitamin D per day for eight weeks; and also take an extra 5,000 IU pill every Monday, Wednesday, and Friday (so you would take a total of 10,000 units on those three days). This gives the same total of 50,000 IU per week. Some patients find the daily dose easier to remember.

Both ways work well, and some of my patients prefer the daily route rather than trying to remember a specific day of the week when they are supposed to take their vitamin D. My preference in general is to encourage my patients to take the vitamin D daily along with their other daily supplements.

After eight weeks, I measure their level again. Depending on a patient's individual biochemistry, the vitamin D supplement may have only brought the level up to 25 to 30 ng/ml. If this is the case, I then give the patient another eight weeks of 50,000 IU per week. At the end of that period, I repeat the blood test again and almost everyone, no matter how low the starting values were, will be over 40 ng/ml at that point. They then go on a maintenance dose of vitamin D, which in my practice is now 2,000 IU/day.

The subject of maintenance doses, just like minimal blood levels, is a hot topic among vitamin D researchers. Some experts recommend 1,000 IU/day, while others recommend up to 4,000 IU/day. One study found that an average man "uses" 3,000 to 4,000 IU/day. I suspect that in time, the normal maintenance dose will become 3,000 to 4,000 IU/day, but it is not yet supported by medical literature. More research needs to be done to confirm the data and to also investigate the dosage in women before I would recommend anyone taking that much on a daily basis without being monitored with regular blood tests.

2. If my patients' blood test shows their 25D level to be between 20 and 30 ng/ml: I do the exact same eight-week protocol as above, recognizing that the patient will probably not need a second round of treatment before going on maintenance therapy.

3. If my patients' blood test shows their 25D level to be between 30 and 40 ng/ml: I again follow the same protocol that I have already described, having my patients take 50,000 IU of vitamin D per week. Because their 25D level is already "normal," according to the current medical literature, they will only take the 50,000 IU for six weeks before I repeat the blood test. After six weeks, we will proceed according to the resulting level, until their blood levels reach 40 ng/ml.

4. If my patients' blood test shows their 25D level to be over 40 ng/ml: I consider this normal and optimized, as do most vitamin D researchers. At this point, I use my clinical judgment to determine treatment. If the patient is a healthy person who has just come for a routine physical, and it is during the summer and they are spending time outside in the sun, I may not recommend vitamin D pills until autumn. Then I will start the patient on 2,000 IU/day.

For patients who have a vitamin D–related health condition, I try to keep their levels between 50 and 70 ng/ml. If needed, I have them take 50,000 IU a week for a while and follow their levels until I get them in that range. Then I put them on a maintenance dose of 2,000 IU/day and watch their blood levels over time. To keep them in that range, however, some patients need up to 4,000 IU per day.

Of course, in all my patients who are taking a maintenance dose, I continue to recommend that they get tested at least once (in March or April) and preferably twice a year (the second time in October or November). A vitamin D test is a routine part of my blood evaluation of every new patient regardless of the time of year, just like a cholesterol or anemia test.

If You Do Not Take a Blood Test to Determine Your Ideal Dose

For those who do not want to get a blood test—either with their doctor or through a home test kit—there are basic doses of vitamin D that I recommend to my patients.

The recommended dose of vitamin D by the Institute of Medicine's Food and Nutrition Board (FNB) is a mere 200 IU/day from birth until 50 years of age for males and females. From 50 to 70 years old, the FNB recommends 400 IU/day, and for people over 70, they recommend 600 IU.

It is the widespread opinion of all leading vitamin D researchers that these recommendations were based on old data from several decades ago, which was only meant to provide the amount of vitamin D necessary to prevent rickets and other bone diseases. With all the new information of the last ten years that I have discussed, vitamin D advocates have realized that the bone benefits are just the tip of the iceberg. All of the other positive effects for the more than 26 vitamin D–responsive tissues in the body require a much higher amount of vitamin D to activate their functions. The top researchers in this field are actively working with the FNB to increase the minimum daily amount recommended. Please see the Appendix at the end of this book to read the call-to-action statement that 14 vitamin D scientists have signed in support of this goal.

Based upon review of the medical literature and discussions I have had with some of the leading vitamin D researchers, I currently recommend the following dosages to my patients and their friends and family members who do not get a blood test:

- **Neonates up to age 1:** 400 IU/day (and possibly more if they are nursing)
- **Ages 1 to 12:** 1,000–2,000 IU/day, depending on weight
- **Children over 12 and all adults:** 2,000 IU/day

I consider these dosages to be conservative and absolutely safe in light of all the available medical literature. I also expect these numbers to rise significantly in the coming months and years, as more and more researchers use higher doses to study the benefits of vitamin D.

There are even several published articles citing the safety of giving newborns 1,000 to 2,000 IU/day with no ill effects. As mentioned earlier there are calls in medical journals for the basic dose for adults to be in the 3,000 to 4,000 IU range per day, and several of my integrative-medicine colleagues are using these doses already. I would only recommend this dosage range if blood tests are followed regularly.

Vitamin D Toxicity

I have already explained that it is actually difficult to become vitamin D toxic, and in medical school I learned that one can overdose because vitamin D is fat soluble. It was made to sound as if overdoses were common and easy to achieve. In point of fact, this is not true.

With patients who are getting all their vitamin D from sunshine, their skin has protective mechanisms to prevent toxicity. Once the level is elevated, their skin will "sidetrack" the excess into pathways that break it down. However, in light of the fact that vitamin D pills are now easily available over the counter and on the Internet in doses anywhere from 200 IU to 50,000 IU, the concern over toxicity takes on more significance.

The initial signs of a vitamin D overdose are silent. It starts with an elevated calcium level in urine, and then there is an increased amount of calcium in the blood. A patient might not experience any indication of overdose until significant symptoms have developed. Symptoms of elevated calcium in the blood can include abdominal pain, constipation, muscle weakness, itching, vomiting, and extreme thirst. It can also predispose the patient to kidney stones and high blood pressure.

Much has been written in the medical literature about the levels of vitamin D in the blood that would indicate toxicity. Current data support the viewpoint that the 25-hydroxy D level must be above 150 ng/ml to produce toxicity. However, it is considered more prudent to set the upper limit to 100 ng/ml in order to ensure a wide safety margin. This is what I tell my patients as well, and is also why I conduct blood tests to monitor patients' levels at least once a year. With the vitamin D level of so many people hovering around 20 ng/ml, it would take a lot to produce toxicity.

Current medical literature indicates that an amount of vitamin D in excess of 10,000 IU per day would have to be taken for many months to produce true toxicity. This is obviously very unlikely. There is one case reported in which a patient was taking over 150,000 IU of vitamin D per day for two years. When admitted to the hospital, his vitamin D blood level was over 500 ng/ml. But after a few days of supportive treatment to lower his calcium, he was discharged (and taken off his vitamin D supplement with advice to also avoid the sun). He was monitored as an outpatient, and all of his blood tests returned to normal.

In summary, it is hard to overdose on vitamin D. And certainly with the dosages that I have recommended to my patients, it is extremely unlikely that there would ever be a problem of overdose in an otherwise healthy person.

When Not to Take Vitamin D— or When to Take a Lower Dose

Vitamin D is normally very well tolerated by all people. I could not find any reports in PubMed (an archive of biomedical and life-sciences journals maintained by the U.S. National Institutes of Health) of allergic reactions to vitamin D supplements. However, care should be used in giving vitamin D to patients who have what are known as granulomatous diseases, which includes tuberculosis and sarcoidosis—and now many doctors also count Lyme disease in this category. In addition, vitamin D is not safe for most patients with lymphomas.

Questions have been raised about withholding vitamin D from patients with tuberculosis because they are likely to be significantly deficient in it. Two recent studies have actually shown that giving vitamin D to tuberculosis (TB) patients was helpful in both treating the disease and preventing elevated calcium. This type of benefit is expected in light of the new knowledge about how vitamin D increases antiviral, antibacterial, and antiparasitic immune factors. Vitamin D in the white cells of TB patients has been shown to make a substance called cathelicidin, which can kill TB cells. Current medical literature recommends that patients with granulomatous diseases, like TB, should keep their vitamin D level between 20 and 30 ng/ml.

In addition, an elevated calcium level in the blood can also be a contraindication to vitamin D supplementation. This problem is unusual but should be carefully evaluated by a physician to understand the cause of the raised calcium. Benign tumors of the parathyroid glands can be a cause of this, but it is an uncommon condition.

Another situation in which doctors need to be careful in giving vitamin D is in patients who are taking a drug called hydrochlorothiazide, a mild diuretic commonly used to treat high blood pressure. The reason for caution is because the hydrochlorothiazide itself can raise serum calcium and taking vitamin D could raise it even more, causing kidney stones.

On the other side of the coin, several of the drugs used to treat seizure disorders can cause a vitamin D deficiency. In addition, cimetidine, steroids, and certain asthma medications and weight-loss drugs can lower vitamin D levels. Patients who take these should have their vitamin D level tested regularly.

Vitamin D Dosages and the Stages of Your Life

Vitamin D Dosages During Pregnancy

Vitamin D deficiency in pregnant women is near epidemic proportions in the U.S. and in most of the world. One study by J.M. Lee, M.D., Ph.D., and others found that 50 percent of mothers and 65 percent of their newborns were vitamin D deficient although most of the mothers took a prenatal vitamin with D in it.

The fetus uses the mother's vitamin D and, therefore, requirements for vitamin D during pregnancy increase. Vitamin D concentrations in the mother will tend to fall during the third trimester. This is especially true if that part of the pregnancy is occurring during the winter. At the time of birth, studies show that 25D in the umbilical cord at delivery is approximately 80 percent of the mother's blood level.

Severe deficiency during pregnancy can, of course, lead to rickets in the newborn due to the decrease in the mineralization of the baby's skeleton. In another study, it was shown that the higher the 25D level of the mother, the lower the likelihood of her developing preeclampsia. Studies in animals continue to show that vitamin D deficiency permanently injures the fetus's brain.

Research clearly illustrates that the current recommendation of 400 IU/day is insufficient during pregnancy and will not significantly raise the umbilical-cord level of vitamin D. Unfortunately, 400 IU is all that is in most prenatal vitamins. A recent study showed that in pregnant women who took 800 IU of vitamin D from week 27 until delivery, the mother's vitamin D level at delivery was still less than 20 ng/ml. Certainly, I would guess the baby's level was also low.

As this book was going to press, a new article about vitamin D and pregnancy was just published. Doctors followed 253 births at a Boston hospital from 2005 to 2007. Once they controlled for other variables, the doctors found that women with very low vitamin D levels (less than 15 ng/ml) were almost four times more likely to have a C-section than women who were not so deficient.

It is my opinion that during pregnancy, women should have their vitamin D level checked approximately every three months and should be treated by their physician to keep their level above 30 ng/ml, and preferably above 40 ng/ml. In some situations, 4,000 or 5,000 IU/day of vitamin D for several weeks may be necessary to normalize the mother's vitamin D so that it is at least above 30 ng/ml.

Vitamin D Dosages for Breast-Fed Infants

As I have mentioned, unfortunately, most human milk contains very little vitamin D (approximately 20 IU per liter). Women who have a vitamin D deficiency will provide even less of it to their infants. There is good evidence to suggest that breast-fed infants who are not supplemented with vitamin D during the first six months of life will have a level below 20 ng/ml and are thus at increased risk to develop rickets.

Studies have shown that women who are exclusively feeding their newborn with breast milk may need to be taking up to 4,000 IU of vitamin D per day. This will not only increase their own level to more than 30 ng/ml, but it will also enable them to transfer enough of it into their milk to meet their child's requirements. As mentioned earlier, if I give a nursing woman this much vitamin D, I follow her blood tests regularly.

An alternative way to meet the child's requirements will be for the nursing mother to take a lower dose of vitamin D for herself and give her newborn 400 IU/day. In Canada, current guidelines recommend that all infants be given this dose every day. I am happy to see that the American Academy of Pediatrics recently doubled their recommendations of vitamin D for infants and children. They now recommend 400 IU per day for all children beginning in the first few days of life. To make this easier, vitamin D now comes as drops that can be put in juice or water.

In contrast, the National Health and Nutrition Examination Survey (NHANES) conducted from 1999 to 2002 found that less than 10 percent of American infants, aged birth to 12 months, were receiving supplemental vitamin D. Clearly this needs to change!

In an ideal world, all mothers should have their own vitamin D levels checked, as I do in my practice, and the babies should have their levels checked, too. The availability of the new home blood-spot test makes checking the child's vitamin D level easy. The vitamin D requirements for newborns are still up in the air in the medical literature now and have not been settled. As I have said earlier, I recommend that newborns be given 400 IU of vitamin D per day, but this may soon go up to 1,000 IU/day. I mentioned that a study was done in sun-starved Finland with more than 10,000 infants given 2,000 IU of vitamin D per day during their first year of life. These children were then followed for 31 years. Their risk of developing type 1 diabetes over those years was reduced by almost 80 percent. There were also no adverse effects reported by taking that dosage of vitamin D.

Many of my patients choose to exclusively nurse their newborns. In this case, I will keep the mother's 25D level over 40 ng/ml. Otherwise, I will ask the mother to give her child 400 IU of vitamin D a day as drops in water or juice. In my opinion, this is the best way to ensure the baby is getting enough vitamin D in their early months of life.

Vitamin D Dosages for Children and Young Adults

In children and young adults, there is also a significant incidence of vitamin D deficiency. In a study conducted in Boston, 52 percent of Hispanic and black adolescents were deficient in vitamin D. In another study in Maine, 48 percent of preadolescent girls had vitamin D levels less than 20 ng/ml. And in studies in Lebanon, Turkey, India, Australia, the United Arab Emirates, and Saudi Arabia, 30 to 50 percent of children had levels less than 20 ng/ml. Furthermore, research has shown that children and young adults who had significant exposure to sunlight had a 40 percent reduction in their risk of non-Hodgkin's lymphoma.

As reported in the NHANES study, American children from one to five years old were found to have an average vitamin D level of only about 22 ng/ml. Without sufficient vitamin D, only approximately one-third of their dietary calcium is absorbed compared to children who have normal levels of vitamin D.

As this book goes to press, the amount that the Institute of Medicine considers to be an adequate intake for children and young adults is only 200 IU. However, most vitamin D experts recommend that without sufficient sun exposure, children from age one and up should take at least 1,000 IU/day of vitamin D. This is what I do in my practice. As children approach their teens, without blood tests, I increase the dosage to 2,000 IU/day.

Ideally, all children will have an occasional blood test done to check their levels. With the new fingerstick test I described earlier, it is now much easier than ever before to get an accurate vitamin D blood test and reading.

In Summary

A simple blood test is the best way to learn what your vitamin D level is. It is easy for your doctor to order this, and now there is even a home self-test you can use to determine your level. I encourage you to test your blood level of vitamin D to find out if this health-enhancing nutrient is at work for you.

I also encourage you to optimize your blood level of vitamin D to 40 ng/ml (or slightly higher).This is done by taking high-quality vitamin D supplements followed by additional testing. I hope I was able to take the mystery and confusion out of this process by describing what has worked in my medical practice.

I hope you feel empowered from all you have learned to participate in your own health care. Once you get started, I believe you will see that the supplementation protocol I recommend to my own patients is very straightforward. May you always have a healthy, active life . . . and optimal vitamin D levels.

Afterword

A NEW VITAMIN D WORLD

Simply stated, my mission is to get every person in the world to have optimal vitamin D levels! As I finish writing this book, there are more than 44,000 articles on vitamin D in PubMed, the major medical search engine—and a search on Google brought up 12 million links! The plethora of articles detailing every nuance of the benefits of vitamin D will continue to pour forth from the research laboratories of the world.

Clearly, awareness of the problem of vitamin D deficiency is increasing rapidly. In this book, I have highlighted and discussed all the major articles and information available today about the numerous benefits of normalizing your vitamin D level as well as your family members' and friends'.

In the years ahead, I expect all the retrospective and epidemiological studies that show the benefits of vitamin D will be further confirmed by prospective randomized-controlled trials. Then, finally, all doctors will be convinced that vitamin D will help their patients. This will also be taught in medical schools throughout the world. The medical community will have more clarity on optimal dosages for cancer patients, pregnant women, newborns, and for every man and woman.

To paraphrase John Lennon, imagine a world where all these answers were already known, where everybody was taking vitamin D. What would that world look like? What would happen to the incidence rates of cancer? What would happen to heart attack and stroke rates? What would the prevalence of juvenile diabetes look like? Or autoimmune diseases? Or autism?

What would the effects be if we normalized the vitamin D levels of all the people on the continent of Africa where infectious diseases are rampant? How would normalizing vitamin D levels in every patient with HIV/AIDS affect their prognosis? What would be the outcome of normalizing the vitamin D levels of the children and adults of rural America? You may say that I am a dreamer, but that is the world I see in my mind's eye, and it is the world I want you to help me bring about.

Talk to Your Friends and Relatives

If you are as convinced about the benefits of vitamin D as I am, why don't you give all of your friends and relatives a gift of a bottle of vitamin D_3 (2,000 IU), and ask them to start taking one a day? Tell them to get their children, and especially their newborns, on vitamin D supplements. Ask all of your friends who are pregnant to take extra vitamin D, particularly while nursing. I have very clearly outlined the dosages that I have been safely recommending to my patients for years. Imagine the benefits that taking vitamin D could bring to your family and friends. As I have demonstrated throughout the book, such dosages will cause absolutely no harm.

Talk to Your Doctor

Help me bring awareness to all the physicians of the world about the importance of vitamin D for their patients. Perhaps you will buy a copy of this book as a gift for your doctor.

Of course, your doctor may be skeptical at first, especially when hearing that you are taking doses of vitamin D in the thousands. This is because physicians were educated about vitamin D based on information from several decades ago. Help your doctor know that 2,000 IU of vitamin D is only 50 micrograms.

In particular, I would like to give you two references that will be easy for your physician to review. The first is a recent classic article on vitamin D deficiency by the world famous Dr. Michael Holick:

"Vitamin D Deficiency," by Michael Holick, M.D., Ph.D.
New England Journal of Medicine 2007; volume 357, pages 266–81

The second is another classic article on vitamin D deficiency by Dr. John Cannell and others. The reference for your doctor is:

"Diagnosis and Treatment of Vitamin D Deficiency," by J.J. Cannell, M.D., et al.
Expert Opinion Pharmacotherapy 2008; volume 9, issue 1, pages 1–12

You can copy this page of the book and give your doctor these exact references.

Encouraging your doctors to read recent studies on vitamin D and eventually prescribe it on a daily basis in their practice can help thousands of people in your community, and this can spread throughout the world.

◨◼◨

It is hard to put this book to bed—a publisher's term for finishing a book. By the time you have read this, many more vitamin D studies will have been published with more information, recommendations, and even more exciting news.

Fortunately, we have the Internet today. As I have mentioned, I intend to maintain an active dialogue with frequent updates on vitamin D as new studies come out. Be sure to regularly visit the Website connected with this book: **www.VitaminDRevolution.com**.

I also invite you to communicate with me in the Website's blog so that we may have a discussion that spills over to millions of people. In this way, we can create a higher level of health for the whole world through the use of this amazing hormone we call vitamin D.

Until we meet again . . . namaste.

Appendix

VITAMIN D SCIENTISTS' CALL-TO-ACTION STATEMENT

We are aware of substantial scientific evidence supporting the role of vitamin D in prevention of cancer. It has been reasonably established that adequate serum vitamin D metabolite levels are associated with substantially lower incidence rates of several types of cancer, including those of the breast, colon, and ovary, and other sites.

We have concluded that the vitamin D status of most individuals in North America will need to be greatly improved for substantial reduction in incidence of cancer. Epidemiological studies have shown that higher vitamin D levels are also associated with lower risk of Type I diabetes in children and of multiple sclerosis. Several studies have found that markers of higher vitamin D levels are associated with lower incidence and severity of influenza and several other infectious diseases.

Higher vitamin D status can be achieved in part by increased oral intake of vitamin D_3. The appropriate intake of vitamin D_3 for cancer risk reduction depends on the individual's age, race, lifestyle, and latitude of residence. New evidence indicates that the intake should be 2000 IU per day. Intake of 2000 IU/day is the current upper limit of the National Academy of Sciences, Institute of Medicine, Food and Nutrition Board. New evidence also indicates that the upper limit should be raised substantially. The levels that are needed to prevent a substantial proportion of cancer would also be effective in substantially reducing risk of fractures, Type I childhood diabetes, and multiple sclerosis.

Greater oral intakes of vitamin D_3 may be needed in the aged and in individuals who spend little time outdoors, because of reduced cutaneous synthesis. Choice of a larger dose may be based on the individual's wintertime serum 25(OH)D level.

For those choosing to have serum 25-hydroxyvitamin D tested, a target serum level should be chosen in consultation with a health care provider, based on the characteristics of the individual. An approximate guideline for health care providers who choose to measure serum 25-hydroxyvitamin D in their patients would aim for 40–60 ng/ml, unless there are specific contraindications. Contraindications are extremely rare, and are well known to physicians. No intervention is free of all risk, including this one. Patients should be advised of this, and advised in detail of risks that may be specific to the individual.

Any risks of vitamin D inadequacy considerably exceed any risks of taking 2000 IU/day of vitamin D_3, which the NAS-IOM regards as having no adverse health effect.

A substantially higher level of support for research on the role of vitamin D for the prevention of cancer is urgently needed. However, delays in taking reasonable preventive action on cancer by ensuring nearly universal oral intake of vitamin D_3 of 2000 IU/day is costing thousands of lives unnecessarily each year that are lost due to fractures, cancer, diabetes, multiple sclerosis, and other diseases for which vitamin D deficiency plays a major role.

Updated April 30, 2008

Scientists

John J. Cannell, M.D.
Atascadero State Hospital

Cedric F. Garland, Dr. P.H.
F.A.C.E.
University of California San Diego

Frank C. Garland, Ph.D.
University of California San Diego

Edward Giovannucci, M.D., Sc.D
Harvard School of Public Health

Edward D. Gorham, M.P.H., Ph.D.
University of California San Diego

William B. Grant, Ph.D.
Sunlight, Nutrition, and Health
Research Center (SUNARC)

John Hathcock, Ph.D.
Council for Responsible Nutrition

Robert P. Heaney, M.D.
Creighton University

Michael F. Holick, Ph.D., M.D.
Boston University School of
Medicine

Bruce W. Hollis, Ph.D.
Medical University of South
Carolina

Joan M. Lappe, Ph.D., R.N.
F.A.A.N.
Creighton University

Anthony W. Norman, Ph.D.
University of California Riverside

Reinhold Vieth, Ph.D. F.C.A.C.B.
University of Toronto
Mount Sinai Hospital

Walter C. Willett, Dr. P.H., M.D.
Harvard School of Public Health

GrassrootsHealth
A Public Health Promotion Organization

□□■ ■□□

Glossary

Activated vitamin D: Also known as $1,25D_3$ or calcitriol, this form of vitamin D is a steroid hormone. It is fat soluble and can pass through cell membranes to bind to the vitamin D receptors. It is a very powerful steroid hormone, and it regulates gene expression by being able to switch on and off approximately 200 genes in the body.

Angioneogenesis: The process of creating new blood vessels. Cancer cells do this to support their growth.

Apoptosis: A type of programmed cell death. Cancer cells lose the ability to program death, which helps them grow uncontrollably.

Autocrine: The process whereby a cell makes its own chemical messenger (in this case, activated vitamin D) that binds to receptors inside the same cell and leads to changes in the biochemical functioning of the cell.

Blood level: The amount of vitamin D in the form of 25D (calcidiol) that circulates in the blood. It is measured in nanograms per milliliter (ng/ml). (An alternate measure is nanomoles per litre, or nmol/L.) According to literature referenced in this book, the current "normal" levels for 25D are above 30 ng/ml with 40 to 70 ng/ml being optimal. Vitamin D blood levels should be tested with a 25-hydroxyvitamin D blood test.

Bone mineral density (BMD): The amount of mineral content (calcium) in the bone.

Calcidiol: Also known as 25D in this book. It is a prehormone made from vitamin D_3 in the blood. This is the form of vitamin D that is tested with a 25-hydroxyvitamin D blood test.

Calcitriol: See *activated vitamin D*.

Calcium: A mineral necessary for the development of healthy bones. Adequate levels of vitamin D are necessary to facilitate calcium absorption.

Cholecalciferol: Known as vitamin D_3 in this book, it is the raw material from which all potent forms of vitamin D are produced in the body. It is naturally produced in the skin of humans and animals when UVB sunlight hits the skin.

Congestive heart failure (CHF): A weakened condition of the heart muscle, impairing its ability to pump blood.

Diabetes mellitus: A metabolic disorder, characterized by excess glucose in the blood. It is usually caused by insufficient insulin to carry the glucose into the cells.

Endocrine: The system in the body whereby one organ will secrete a molecule (such as a hormone) into the bloodstream or lymphatic system, which has an effect on another distant organ in a different part of the body.

Epidemic: An outbreak of illness or disease affecting a large number of people at the same time at unexpected rates.

Epidemiological: Used to refer to studies that look at the distribution, incidence, and cause of disease in specific populations.

Ergocalciferol: Also known as vitamin D_2, it is a form of vitamin D manufactured from plants and fungi. It does not occur naturally in humans and is significantly less potent than naturally occurring vitamin D_3. This form of vitamin D is not recommended for the optimization of vitamin D levels.

Hypertension: Another term for high blood pressure.

Immune system: The body's complex mechanism of cells and organs that serve to protect the body from infection with bacteria, parasites, and viruses.

International unit (IU): A unit of measurement is an accepted standard based on the biological activity of the substance. The IU for vitamin D is unique to this substance—for example, 100 IU of vitamin D does not equal 100 IU of vitamin E. One thousand IU of vitamin D equals 0.025 milligrams (mg) or 25 micrograms (mcg) of vitamin D.

Macrophage: A type of white blood cell that is an important part of the immune response, helping to destroy protozoa, bacteria, and cancer cells.

Malignant: Usually used as a synonym for cancer—as in a "malignant tumor."

Maximum upper limit: An amount set by the government as the recommended maximum levels of a substance to be taken with the intention of eliminating the possibility of any negative health effects.

Metastasis: Describes the spread of cancer cells through the bloodstream or lymphatic system into other tissues and organs.

Minimal erythemal dose (MED): The amount of sun or UV exposure necessary to turn the skin pink.

Multiple sclerosis (MS): A degenerative, most likely, autoimmune disease that affects the central nervous system—specifically, the myelin that protects the brain and the spinal cord.

Nanograms/milliliter (ng/ml): One unit of measurement for the amount of activated vitamin D in the blood.

Nanomoles/litre (nmol/L): Another unit of measurement for the amount of activated vitamin D in the blood. To convert ng/ml to nmol/L, multiply by 2.5 (for example, 40 ng/ml = 100 nmol/L).

Neuromuscular: Having to do with both the nerves and the muscle tissue.

NHANES: National Health and Nutrition Examination Surveys designed to gather health and nutritional information from people in the U.S. for the purpose of medical research and improving the health of the country.

Osteomalacia: Known as adult rickets. When adult bones rebuild, they do not harden properly, resulting in weaker, softer bones. Osteomalacia is associated with deep musculoskeletal pain and can often be mistaken for fibromyalgia.

Osteoporosis: A disease in which the bones do not rebuild as fast as they are broken down, resulting in weak, porous bones that are susceptible to fracture. A fracture may be the first indication of this painless disease.

Prehormone: A substance secreted by the glands that has little or no biological activity by itself, and is later converted into an actual hormone.

Recommended daily allowance (RDA): The amount of a nutrient that is deemed necessary to maintain health. The recommendations are made by the Food and Nutrition Board, a unit of the Institute of Medicine, which is part of The National Academy of Sciences. The amounts recommended are intended to meet the nutritional requirements of the vast majority of the healthy population of the U.S.

Seasonal affective disorder (SAD): A form of depression that occurs seasonally in the winter months and is associated with low levels of sunlight. It is sometimes referred to as the "winter blues." Other symptoms of SAD include anxiety, fatigue, headaches, and sleep problems.

Secosteroid: A molecule that has a similar structure to a steroid. Vitamin D is our body's most important secosteroid.

7-dehydrocholesterol: A type of cholesterol molecule in the skin that allows the skin to make vitamin D_3 from the UVB rays in sunlight.

Steroid hormone: An important type of hormone that can stimulate receptor molecules and affect gene expression. Steroid molecules have a specific molecular structure that qualifies them to be a steroid.

Tuberculosis (TB): A contagious, potentially fatal disease caused by bacteria that usually invades the lungs.

Ultraviolet A (UVA): The long rays from the sun, which do not cause sunburn, but do penetrate more deeply into the skin and contribute to premature aging, discoloration, and wrinkles.

Ultraviolet B (UVB): The rays responsible for turning skin red and causing sunburn. When UVB rays hit the skin, they launch the production of vitamin D.

Vitamin D: A substance produced naturally in the body when skin is exposed to UVB rays. Vitamin D has been associated with the functioning of organs, tissues, and bones, as well as the metabolism of calcium and phosphorus in the body.

Vitamin D$_2$: See *ergocalciferol*.

Vitamin D$_3$: See *cholecalciferol*.

Vitamin D level: See *blood level*.

Vitamin D receptor (VDR): Most tissues and organs in the body have vitamin D receptors, giving them the ability to metabolize 25D into activated vitamin D.

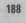

Bibliography

References Chapter One

Cannell JJ, Hollis BW. Use of vitamin D in clinical practice. *Altern Med Rev.* 2008 Mar;13(1):6-20. PMID: 18377099

Holick MF, Chen TC. Vitamin D deficiency: a worldwide problem with health consequences. *Am J Clin Nutr.* 2008 Apr;87(4):1080S-6S. Review. PMID: 18400738

Holick MF. Vitamin D deficiency. *N Engl J Med.* 2007 Jul 19;357(3):266-81. Review. No abstract available. PMID: 17634462

Norman AW. From vitamin D to hormone D: fundamentals of the vitamin D endocrine system essential for good health. *Am J Clin Nutr.* 2008 Aug;88(2):491S-499S. Review. PMID: 18689389

Schwartz GG, Whitlatch LW, Chen TC, Lokeshwar BL, Holick MF. Human prostate cells synthesize 1,25-dihydroxyvitamin D3 from 25-hydroxyvitamin D3. *Cancer Epidemiol Biomarkers Prev.* 1998 May;7(5):391-5. PMID: 9610788

Wortsman J, Matsuoka LY, Chen TC, Lu Z, Holick MF. Decreased bioavailability of vitamin D in obesity. *Am J Clin Nutr.* 2000 Sep;72(3):690-3. Erratum in: *Am J Clin Nutr.* 2003 May;77(5):1342. PMID: 10966885

References Chapter Two

Bertone-Johnson ER. Prospective studies of dietary vitamin D and breast cancer: more questions raised than answered. *Nutr Rev.* 2007 Oct;65(10):459-66. Review. PMID: 17972440

Cannell JJ, Hollis BW, Zasloff M, Heaney RP. Diagnosis and treatment of vitamin D deficiency. *Expert Opin Pharmacother.* 2008 Jan;9(1):107-18. PMID: 18076342

Dowd, James, and Stafford, Dianne, *The Vitamin D Cure.* John Wiley & Sons. 2008

Giovannucci E, Liu Y, Hollis BW, Rimm EB. 25-hydroxyvitamin D and risk of myocardial infarction in men: a prospective study. *Arch Intern Med.* 2008 Jun 9;168(11):1174-80. PMID: 18541825

Holick MF. Vitamin D deficiency. *N Engl J Med.* 2007 Jul 19;357(3):266-81. Review. No abstract available. PMID: 17634462

Holick MF. Sunlight and vitamin D for bone health and prevention of autoimmune diseases, cancers, and cardiovascular disease. *Am J Clin Nutr.* 2004 Dec;80(6 Suppl):1678S-88S. Review. PMID: 15585788

Holick MF. *The UV Advantage.* Simon & Shuster. 2003

References Chapter Three

Cannell JJ, Hollis BW. Use of vitamin D in clinical practice. *Altern Med Rev.* 2008 Mar;13(1):6-20. PMID: 18377099

Cannell JJ, Hollis BW, Zasloff M, Heaney RP. Diagnosis and treatment of vitamin D deficiency. *Expert Opin Pharmacother.* 2008 Jan;9(1):107-18. PMID: 18076342

Dawson-Hughes B. Serum 25-hydroxyvitamin D and functional outcomes in the elderly. *Am J Clin Nutr.* 2008 Aug;88(2):537S-540S. Review. PMID: 18689397

Grant WB, Holick MF. Benefits and requirements of vitamin D for optimal health: a review. *Altern Med Rev.* 2005 Jun;10(2):94-111. Review. PMID: 15989379

Grant WB. An estimate of premature cancer mortality in the U.S. due to inadequate doses of solar ultraviolet-B radiation. *Cancer.* 2002 Mar 15;94(6):1867-75. PMID: 11920550

Greer FR. 25-Hydroxyvitamin D: functional outcomes in infants and young children. *Am J Clin Nutr.* 2008 Aug;88(2):529S-533S. Review. PMID: 18689395

Holick MF. Vitamin D deficiency. *N Engl J Med.* 2007 Jul 19;357(3):266-81. Review. No abstract available. PMID: 17634462

Holick MF. Vitamin D deficiency: what a pain it is. *Mayo Clin Proc.* 2003 Dec;78(12):1457-9. No abstract available. PMID: 14661673

Holick MF. *The UV Advantage.* Simon & Shuster. 2003

Kovacs CS. Vitamin D in pregnancy and lactation: maternal, fetal, and neonatal outcomes from human and animal studies. *Am J Clin Nutr.* 2008 Aug;88(2):520S-528S. Review. PMID: 18689394

Macdonald HM, Mavroeidi A, Barr RJ, Black AJ, Fraser WD, Reid DM. Vitamin D status in postmenopausal women living at higher latitudes in the UK in relation to bone health, overweight, sunlight exposure and dietary vitamin D. *Bone*. 2008 May;42(5):996-1003. Epub 2008 Feb 9. PMID: 18329355

References Chapter Four

Adams, M. *The Healing Power of Sunlight and Vitamin D: An Exclusive Interview with Dr. Michael Holick*. Truth Publishing International, Ltd. 2005

Al Faraj S, Al Mutairi K. Vitamin D deficiency and chronic low back pain in Saudi Arabia. *Spine*. 2003 Jan 15;28(2):177-9. PMID: 12544936

Baker K, Zhang YQ, Goggins J, et al. Hypovitaminosis D and its association with muscle strength, pain and physical function in knee osteoarthritis (OA): a 30-month longitudinal, observational study [abstract]. Presented at the 66th Annual Scientific Meeting of the American College of Rheumatology; October 17-21, 2004; San Antonio, Texas

Cannell JJ, Hollis BW. Use of vitamin D in clinical practice. *Altern Med Rev*. 2008 Mar;13(1):6-20. PMID: 18377099

Cannell JJ, Hollis BW, Zasloff M, Heaney RP. Diagnosis and treatment of vitamin D deficiency. *Expert Opin Pharmacother*. 2008 Jan;9(1):107-18. PMID: 18076342

Cannell JJ, Vieth R, Umhau JC, Holick MF, Grant WB, Madronich S, Garland CF, Giovannucci E. Epidemic influenza and vitamin D. *Epidemiol Infect.* 2006 Dec;134(6):1129-40. Epub 2006 Sep 7. Review. PMID: 16959053

Crew, KD, et al. High prevalence of vitamin D deficiency in a multi-ethnic cohort of premenopausal breast cancer patients. *J Clin Oncol* 26: 2008 (May 20 suppl; abstr 9583).

Dawson-Hughes B. Serum 25-hydroxyvitamin D and functional outcomes in the elderly. *Am J Clin Nutr.* 2008 Aug;88(2):537S-540S. Review. PMID: 18689397

Dietrich T, Joshipura KJ, Dawson-Hughes B, Bischoff-Ferrari HA. Association between serum concentrations of 25-hydroxyvitamin D_3 and periodontal disease in the US population. *Am J Clin Nutr.* 2004 Jul;80(1):108-13. PMID: 15213036

Dowd, James, and Stafford, Dianne. *The Vitamin D Cure.* John Wiley & Sons. 2008.

Garland CF, Gorham ED, Mohr SB, Grant WB, Giovannucci EL, Lipkin M, Newmark H, Holick MF, Garland FC. Vitamin D and prevention of breast cancer: pooled analysis. *J Steroid Biochem Mol Biol.* 2007 Mar;103(3-5):708-11. PMID: 17368188

Giovannucci E, Liu Y, Hollis BW, Rimm EB. 25-hydroxyvitamin D and risk of myocardial infarction in men: a prospective study. *Arch Intern Med.* 2008 Jun 9;168(11):1174-80. PMID: 18541825

Gorham ED, Garland CF, Garland FC, Grant WB, Mohr SB, Lipkin M, Newmark HL, Giovannucci E, Wei M, Holick MF. Optimal vitamin D status for colorectal cancer prevention: a quantitative meta analysis. *Am J Prev Med*. 2007 Mar;32(3):210-6. PMID: 17296473

Grant WB, Holick MF. Benefits and requirements of vitamin D for optimal health: a review. *Altern Med Rev*. 2005 Jun;10(2):94-111. Review. PMID: 15989379

Heaney RP. Long-latency deficiency disease: insights from calcium and vitamin D. *Am J Clin Nutr*. 2003 Nov;78(5):912-9. Review. PMID: 14594776

Holick MF. Calcium plus vitamin D and the risk of colorectal cancer. *N Engl J Med*. 2006 May 25;354(21):2287-8. PMID: 16723623

Holick MF. Vitamin D and sunlight: strategies for cancer prevention and other health benefits. *Clin J Am Soc Nephrol*. 2008 Sep;3(5):1548-54. Epub 2008 Jun 11. PMID: 18550652

Holick MF, Chen TC. Vitamin D deficiency: a worldwide problem with health consequences. *Am J Clin Nutr*. 2008 Apr;87(4):1080S-6S. Review. PMID: 18400738

Holick MF. Vitamin D deficiency. *N Engl J Med*. 2007 Jul 19;357(3):266-81. Review. No abstract available. PMID: 17634462

Holick MF. Vitamin D: importance in the prevention of cancers, type 1 diabetes, heart disease, and osteoporosis. *Am J Clin Nutr*. 2004 Mar;79(3):362-71. Review. Erratum in: *Am J Clin Nutr*. 2004 May;79(5):890. PMID: 14985208

Holick MF. Vitamin D deficiency: what a pain it is. *Mayo Clin Proc.* 2003 Dec;78(12):1457-9. No abstract available. PMID: 14661673

Holick MF. *The UV Advantage*. Simon & Shuster. 2003

Hope-Simpson RE. *The Transmission of Epidemic Influenza*. New York: Plenum Press, 1992.

Houston DK, Cesari M, Ferrucci L, Cherubini A, Maggio D, Bartali B, Johnson MA, Schwartz GG, Kritchevsky SB. Association between vitamin D status and physical performance: the InCHIANTI study. *J Gerontol A Biol Sci Med Sci.* 2007 Apr;62(4):440-6. PMID: 17452740

Houston DK, Cesari M, Ferrucci L, Cherubini A, Maggio D, Bartali B, Johnson MA, Schwartz GG, Kritchevsky SB. Association between vitamin D status and physical performance: the InCHIANTI study. *J Gerontol A Biol Sci Med Sci.* 2007 Apr;62(4):440-6. PMID: 17452740

Hyppönen E, Läärä E, Reunanen A, Järvelin MR, Virtanen SM. Intake of vitamin D and risk of type 1 diabetes: a birth-cohort study. *Lancet.* 2001 Nov 3;358(9292):1500-3. PMID: 11705562

Lappe JM, Travers-Gustafson D, Davies KM, Recker RR, Heaney RP. Vitamin D and calcium supplementation reduces cancer risk: results of a randomized trial. *Am J Clin Nutr.* 2007 Jun;85(6):1586-91. Erratum in: *Am J Clin Nutr.* 2008 Mar;87(3):794. PMID: 17556697

Leavitt, SB. A Neglected "Analgesic" for Chronic Musculoskeletal Pain An Evidence-Based Review & Clinical Practice Guidance. *Pain Treatment Topics*, June 2008

Lee P, Chen R. Vitamin D as an analgesic for patients with type 2 diabetes and neuropathic pain. *Arch Intern Med.* 2008 Apr 14;168(7):771-2. No abstract available. PMID: 18413561

Mohr SB, Garland CF, Gorham ED, Garland FC. The association between ultraviolet B irradiance, vitamin D status and incidence rates of type 1 diabetes in 51 regions worldwide. *Diabetologia.* 2008 Aug;51(8):1391-8. Epub 2008 Jun 12. PMID: 18548227

Mohr SB, Garland CF, Gorham ED, Grant WB, Garland FC. Could ultraviolet B irradiance and vitamin D be associated with lower incidence rates of lung cancer? *J Epidemiol Community Health.* 2008 Jan;62(1):69-74. PMID: 18079336

Neuhouser ML, Sorensen B, Hollis BW, et al. Vitamin D insufficiency in a multiethnic cohort of breast cancer survivors. *Am J Clin Nutr.* 2008 Jul;88(1):133-9. PMID: 18614733

Ng K, Meyerhardt JA, Wu K, Feskanich D, Hollis BW, Giovannucci EL, Fuchs CS. Circulating 25-hydroxyvitamin d levels and survival in patients with colorectal cancer. *J Clin Oncol.* 2008 Jun 20;26(18):2984-91. PMID: 18565885

Pittas AG, Lau J, Hu FB, Dawson-Hughes B. The role of vitamin D and calcium in type 2 diabetes. A systematic review and meta-analysis. *J Clin Endocrinol Metab.* 2007 Jun;92(6):2017-29. Epub 2007 Mar 27. Review. PMID: 17389701

Porojnicu AC, Robsahm TE, Dahlback A, Berg JP, Christiani D, Bruland OS, Moan J. Seasonal and geographical variations in lung cancer prognosis in Norway. Does Vitamin D from the sun play a role? *Lung Cancer.* 2007 Mar;55(3):263-70. Epub 2007 Jan 17. PMID: 17207891

Tuohimaa P, Tenkanen L, et al. Both high and low levels of blood vitamin D are associated with a higher prostate cancer risk: a longitudinal, nested case-control study in the Nordic countries. *Int J Cancer.* 2004 Jan 1;108(1):104-8. PMID: 14618623

Woo TC, Choo R, Jamieson M, Chander S, Vieth R. Pilot study: potential role of vitamin D (Cholecalciferol) in patients with PSA relapse after definitive therapy. *Nutr Cancer.* 2005;51(1):32-6. PMID: 15749627

Vieth R, Kimball S. Vitamin D in congestive heart failure. *Am J Clin Nutr.* 2006 Apr;83(4):731-2. No abstract available. PMID: 16600920

Vieth R, Kimball S, Hu A, Walfish PG. Randomized comparison of the effects of the vitamin D_3 adequate intake versus 100 mcg (4000 IU) per day on biochemical responses and the wellbeing of patients. *Nutr J.* 2004 Jul 19;3:8. PMID: 15260882

Wheeler SD. Vitamin D Deficiency in Chronic Migraine. *Program Abstracts 50th Annual Scientific Meeting American Headache Society* June 26–29, 2008, Boston, MA

Wilkins CH, Sheline YI, Roe CM, Birge SJ, Morris JC. Vitamin D deficiency is associated with low mood and worse cognitive performance in older adults. *Am J Geriatr Psychiatry.* 2006 Dec;14(12):1032-40. PMID: 17138809

Zipitis CS, Akobeng AK. Vitamin D supplementation in early childhood and risk of type 1 diabetes: a systematic review and meta-analysis. *Arch Dis Child.* 2008 Jun;93(6):512-7. Epub 2008 Mar 13. Review. PMID: 18339654

References Chapter Five

Bodnar LM, Catov JM, Simhan HN, Holick MF, Powers RW, Roberts JM. Maternal vitamin D deficiency increases the risk of preeclampsia. *J Clin Endocrinol Metab.* 2007 Sep;92(9):3517-22. Epub 2007 May 29. PMID: 17535985

Cannell, JJ, Vieth, R, Willett, W, et al. Cod liver oil, vitamin A toxicity, frequent respiratory infections, and the vitamin deficiency epidemic. *Annals of Otology, Rhinology & Laryngology.* 2008 117(11):864-870.

Cannell JJ, Hollis BW. Use of vitamin D in clinical practice. *Altern Med Rev.* 2008 Mar;13(1):6-20. PMID: 18377099

Cannell JJ, Hollis BW, Zasloff M, Heaney RP. Diagnosis and treatment of vitamin D deficiency. *Expert Opin Pharmacother.* 2008 Jan;9(1):107-18. PMID: 18076342

Greer FR. 25-Hydroxyvitamin D: functional outcomes in infants and young children. *Am J Clin Nutr.* 2008 Aug;88(2):529S-533S. Review. PMID: 18689395

Holick MF. Vitamin D deficiency. *N Engl J Med.* 2007 Jul 19;357(3):266-81. Review. No abstract available. PMID: 17634462

Hollis BW, Wagner CL, Drezner MK, Binkley NC. Circulating vitamin D_3 and 25-hydroxyvitamin D in humans: An important tool to define adequate nutritional vitamin D status. *J Steroid Biochem Mol Biol.* 2007 Mar;103(3-5):631-4. Epub 2007 Jan 10. PMID: 17218096

Hollis BW, Wagner CL. Vitamin D requirements during lactation: high-dose maternal supplementation as therapy to prevent hypovitaminosis D for both the mother and the nursing infant. *Am J Clin Nutr.* 2004 Dec;80(6 Suppl):1752S-8S. PMID: 15585800

Hyppönen E, Läärä E, Reunanen A, Järvelin MR, Virtanen SM. Intake of vitamin D and risk of type 1 diabetes: a birth-cohort study. *Lancet.* 2001 Nov 3;358(9292):1500-3. PMID: 11705562

Jones G. Pharmacokinetics of vitamin D toxicity. *Am J Clin Nutr.* 2008 Aug;88(2):582S-586S. Review. PMID: 18689406

Kimball S, Fuleihan Gel-H, Vieth R. Vitamin D: a growing perspective. *Crit Rev Clin Lab Sci.* 2008;45(4):339-414. Review. PMID: 18568854

Koutkia P, Chen TC, Holick MF. Vitamin D intoxication associated with an over-the-counter supplement. *N Engl J Med.* 2001 Jul 5;345(1):66-7. No abstract available. PMID: 11439958

Kovacs CS. Vitamin D in pregnancy and lactation: maternal, fetal, and neonatal outcomes from human and animal studies. *Am J Clin Nutr.* 2008 Aug;88(2):520S-528S. Review. PMID: 18689394

Lee JM, Smith JR, Philipp BL, Chen TC, Mathieu J, Holick MF. Vitamin D deficiency in a healthy group of mothers and newborn infants. *Clin Pediatr* (Phila). 2007 Jan;46(1):42-4. PMID: 17164508

Merewood A, Mehta SD, Chen TC, Bauchner H, Holick MF. Association between vitamin D deficiency and primary cesarean section. *J Clin Endocrinol Metab.* 2008 Dec 23. [Epub ahead of print]. PMID: 19106272

Vieth R. The pharmacology of vitamin D, including fortification strategies. In: Feldman D, ed. *Vitamin D*. Vol 2. 2nd ed. Amsterdam, Netherlands: Elsevier Academic Press; 2005:995-1015

Yetley EA. Assessing the vitamin D status of the US population. *Am J Clin Nutr.* 2008 Aug;88(2):558S-564S. Review. PMID: 18689402

References General

Adorini L, Penna G. Control of autoimmune diseases by the vitamin D endocrine system. *Nat Clin Pract Rheumatol.* 2008 Aug;4(8):404-12. Epub 2008 Jul 1. PMID: 18594491

Ahn J, Peters U, et al. Prostate, Lung, Colorectal, and Ovarian Cancer Screening Trial Project Team. Serum vitamin D concentration and prostate cancer risk: a nested case-control study. *J Natl Cancer Inst.* 2008 Jun 4;100(11):796-804. Epub 2008 May 27. PMID: 18505967

Aloia JF, Talwar SA, Pollack S, Feuerman M, Yeh JK. Optimal vitamin D status and serum parathyroid hormone concentrations in African American women. *Am J Clin Nutr.* 2006 Sep;84(3):602-9. PMID: 16960175

Arnson Y, Amital H, Shoenfeld Y. Vitamin D and autoimmunity: new aetiological and therapeutic considerations. *Ann Rheum Dis.* 2007 Sep;66(9):1137-42. Epub 2007 Jun 8. Review. PMID: 17557889

Bao BY, Ting HJ, Hsu JW, Lee YF. Protective role of 1 alpha, 25-dihydroxyvitamin D_3 against oxidative stress in nonmalignant human prostate epithelial cells. *Int J Cancer.* 2008 Jun 15;122(12):2699-706. PMID: 18348143

Boxer RS, Dauser DA, Walsh SJ, Hager WD, Kenny AM. The association between vitamin D and inflammation with the 6-minute walk and frailty in patients with heart failure. *J Am Geriatr Soc.* 2008 Mar;56(3):454-61. Epub 2008 Jan 5. PMID: 18194227

Cannell, JJ, Zasloff, M, et al. On the epidemiology of influenza. *Virology Journal* 2008, 5:29

Cantorna MT, Zhu Y, Froicu M, Wittke A. Vitamin D status, 1,25-dihydroxyvitamin D3, and the immune system. *Am J Clin Nutr.* 2004 Dec;80(6 Suppl):1717S-20S. Review. PMID: 15585793

Chiu KC, Chu A, Go VL, Saad MF. Hypovitaminosis D is associated with insulin resistance and beta cell dysfunction. *Am J Clin Nutr.* 2004 May;79(5):820-5. PMID: 15113720

DeLuca HF. Overview of general physiologic features and functions of vitamin D. *Am J Clin Nutr.* 2004 Dec;80(6 Suppl):1689S-96S. Review. PMID: 15585789

Fosnight SM, Zafirau WJ, Hazelett SE. Vitamin D supplementation to prevent falls in the elderly: evidence and practical considerations. *Pharmacotherapy.* 2008 Feb;28(2):225-34. Review. PMID: 18225968

Garland CF, Grant WB, Mohr SB, Gorham ED, Garland FC. What is the dose-response relationship between vitamin D and cancer risk? *Nutr Rev.* 2007 Aug;65(8 Pt 2):S91-5. Review. PMID: 17867379

Gessner BD, Plotnik J, Muth PT. 25-hydroxyvitamin D levels among healthy children in Alaska. *J Pediatr*. 2003 Oct;143(4):434-7. PMID: 14571215

Goodwin, PJ,. Ennis, M. Frequency of vitamin D (Vit D) deficiency at breast cancer (BC) diagnosis and association with risk of distant recurrence and death in a prospective cohort study of T1-3, N0-1, M0 BC. *J Clin Oncol* 26: 2008 (May 20 suppl; abstr 511)

Grant WB, Garland CF, Gorham ED. An estimate of cancer mortality rate reductions in Europe and the US with 1,000 IU of oral vitamin D per day. *Recent Results Cancer Res*. 2007;174:225-34. Review. PMID: 17302200

Grant WB. Geographic variation of prostate cancer mortality rates in the United States: Implications for prostate cancer risk related to vitamin D. *Int J Cancer*. 2004 Sep 1;111(3):470-1; author reply 472. No abstract available. PMID: 15221981

Heaney RP. Vitamin D in health and disease. *Clin J Am Soc Nephrol*. 2008 Sep;3(5):1535-41. Epub 2008 Jun 4. PMID: 18525006

Heaney RP, Davies KM, Chen TC, Holick MF, Barger-Lux MJ. Human serum 25-hydroxycholecalciferol response to extended oral dosing with cholecalciferol. *Am J Clin Nutr*. 2003 Jan;77(1):204-10. Erratum in: *Am J Clin Nutr*. 2003 Nov;78(5):1047. PMID: 12499343

Hein G, Oelzner P. [Vitamin D metabolites in rheumatoid arthritis: findings--hypotheses--consequences] *Z Rheumatol*. 2000;59 Suppl 1:28-32. German. PMID: 10769432

Holick MF. Deficiency of sunlight and vitamin D. *BMJ*. 2008 Jun 14;336(7657):1318-9. No abstract available. PMID: 18556276

Holick MF, Siris ES, et al. Prevalence of Vitamin D inadequacy among postmenopausal North American women receiving osteoporosis therapy. *J Clin Endocrinol Metab*. 2005 Jun;90(6):3215-24. Epub 2005 Mar 29. PMID: 15797954

Holick MF. Sunlight "D"ilemma: risk of skin cancer or bone disease and muscle weakness. *Lancet*. 2001 Jan 6;357(9249):4-6. No abstract available. PMID: 11197362

Hollis BW, Wagner CL. Vitamin D deficiency during pregnancy: an ongoing epidemic. *Am J Clin Nutr*. 2006 Aug;84(2):273. No abstract available. PMID: 16895872

Hope-Simpson RE, Golubev DB. A new concept of the epidemic process of influenza A virus. *Epidemiol Infect*. 1987 Aug;99(1):5-54. Review. PMID: 3301379

Huisman AM, White KP, Algra A, Harth M, Vieth R, Jacobs JW, Bijlsma JW, Bell DA. Vitamin D levels in women with systemic lupus erythematosus and fibromyalgia. *J Rheumatol*. 2001 Nov;28(11):2535-9. PMID: 11708429

Ingraham BA, Bragdon B, Nohe A. Molecular basis of the potential of vitamin D to prevent cancer. *Curr Med Res Opin*. 2008 Jan;24(1):139-49. Review. PMID: 18034918

Kimball S, Vieth R. Self-prescribed high-dose vitamin D3: effects on biochemical parameters in two men. *Ann Clin Biochem*. 2008 Jan;45(Pt 1):106-10. PMID: 18275686

Lane NE, Gore LR, Cummings SR, Hochberg MC, Scott JC, Williams EN, Nevitt MC. Serum vitamin D levels and incident changes of radiographic hip osteoarthritis: a longitudinal study. *Study of Osteoporotic Fractures Research Group. Arthritis Rheum.* 1999 May;42(5):854-60. PMID: 10323440

Lansdowne AT, Provost SC. Vitamin D$_3$ enhances mood in healthy subjects during winter. *Psychopharmacology* (Berl). 1998 Feb;135(4):319-23. PMID: 9539254

Lee JM, Smith JR, Philipp BL, Chen TC, Mathieu J, Holick MF. Vitamin D deficiency in a healthy group of mothers and newborn infants. *Clin Pediatr* (Phila). 2007 Jan;46(1):42-4. PMID: 17164508

Leslie WD, Miller N, Rogala L, Bernstein CN. Vitamin D status and bone density in recently diagnosed inflammatory bowel disease: the Manitoba IBD Cohort Study. *Am J Gastroenterol.* 2008 Jun;103(6):1451-9. Epub 2008 Apr 16. PMID: 18422819

Litonjua AA, Weiss ST. Is vitamin D deficiency to blame for the asthma epidemic? *J Allergy Clin Immunol.* 2007 Nov;120(5):1031-5. Epub 2007 Oct 24. PMID: 17919705

Luscombe CJ, Fryer AA, French ME, Liu S, Saxby MF, Jones PW, Strange RC. Exposure to ultraviolet radiation: association with susceptibility and age at presentation with prostate cancer. *Lancet.* 2001 Aug 25;358(9282):641-2. PMID: 11530156

McAlindon TE, Felson DT, Zhang Y, Hannan MT, Aliabadi P, Weissman B, Rush D, Wilson PW, Jacques P. Relation of dietary intake and serum levels of vitamin D to progression of osteoarthritis of the knee among participants in the Framingham Study. *Ann Intern Med.* 1996 Sep 1;125(5):353-9. PMID: 8702085

McGrath J, Saari K, Hakko H, Jokelainen J, Jones P, Järvelin MR, Chant D, Isohanni M. Vitamin D supplementation during the first year of life and risk of schizophrenia: a Finnish birth cohort study. *Schizophr Res.* 2004 Apr 1;67(2-3):237-45. PMID: 14984883

Melamed ML, Michos ED, Post W, Astor B. 25-hydroxyvitamin D levels and the risk of mortality in the general population. *Arch Intern Med.* 2008 Aug 11;168(15):1629-37. PMID: 18695076

Merlino LA, Curtis J, Mikuls TR, Cerhan JR, Criswell LA, Saag KG; Iowa Women's Health Study. Vitamin D intake is inversely associated with rheumatoid arthritis: results from the Iowa Women's Health Study. *Arthritis Rheum.* 2004 Jan;50(1):72-7. PMID: 14730601

Moan J, Porojnicu AC, Dahlback A, Setlow RB. Addressing the health benefits and risks, involving vitamin D or skin cancer, of increased sun exposure. *Proc Natl Acad Sci* U S A. 2008 Jan 15;105(2):668-73. Epub 2008 Jan 7. PMID: 18180454

Mohr SB, Garland CF, Gorham ED, Grant WB, Garland FC. Relationship between low ultraviolet B irradiance and higher breast cancer risk in 107 countries. *Breast J.* 2008 May-Jun;14(3):255-60. Epub 2008 Apr 17. PMID: 18422861

Orton SM, Morris AP, Herrera BM, Ramagopalan SV, Lincoln MR, Chao MJ, Vieth R, Sadovnick AD, Ebers GC. Evidence for genetic regulation of vitamin D status in twins with multiple sclerosis. *Am J Clin Nutr.* 2008 Aug;88(2):441-7. PMID: 18689381

Pfeifer M, Begerow B, Minne HW, Nachtigall D, Hansen C. Effects of a short-term vitamin D(3) and calcium supplementation on blood pressure and parathyroid hormone levels in elderly women. *J Clin Endocrinol Metab.* 2001 Apr;86(4):1633-7. PMID: 11297596

Schwalfenberg G. Not enough vitamin D: health consequences for Canadians. *Can Fam Physician.* 2007 May;53(5):841-54. Review. PMID: 17872747

Soltesz G, Patterson CC, Dahlquist G; EURODIAB Study Group. Worldwide childhood type 1 diabetes incidence--what can we learn from epidemiology? *Pediatr Diabetes.* 2007 Oct;8 Suppl 6:6-14. PMID: 17727380

Specker B. Vitamin D requirements during pregnancy. *Am J Clin Nutr.* 2004 Dec;80(6 Suppl):1740S-7S. Review. PMID: 15585798

Szodoray P, Nakken B, Gaal J, Jonsson R, Szegedi A, Zold E, Szegedi G, Brun JG, Gesztelyi R, Zeher M, Bodolay E. The complex role of vitamin D in autoimmune diseases. *Scand J Immunol.* 2008 Sep;68(3):261-9. Epub 2008 May 29. Review. PMID: 18510590

Thys-Jacobs S, Donovan D, Papadopoulos A, Sarrel P, Bilezikian JP. Vitamin D and calcium dysregulation in the polycystic ovarian syndrome. *Steroids.* 1999 Jun;64(6):430-5. PMID: 10433180

van der Meer IM, Karamali NS, Boeke AJ, Lips P, Middelkoop BJ, Verhoeven I, Wuister JD. High prevalence of vitamin D deficiency in pregnant non-Western women in The Hague, Netherlands. *Am J Clin Nutr.* 2006 Aug;84(2):350-3; quiz 468-9. PMID: 16895882

Vasquez A, Manso G, Cannell J. The clinical importance of vitamin D (cholecalciferol): a paradigm shift with implications for all healthcare providers. *Altern Ther Health Med.* 2004 Sep-Oct;10(5):28-36; quiz 37, 94. Review. No abstract available. PMID: 15478784

Visser M, Deeg DJ, Puts MT, Seidell JC, Lips P. Low serum concentrations of 25-hydroxyvitamin D in older persons and the risk of nursing home admission. *Am J Clin Nutr.* 2006 Sep;84(3):616-22; quiz 671-2. PMID: 16960177

Zhou W, Heist RS, et al. Circulating 25-hydroxyvitamin D levels predict survival in early-stage non-small-cell lung cancer patients. *J Clin Oncol.* 2007 Feb 10;25(5):479-85. PMID: 17290055

Zhou W, Suk R, Liu G, Park S, Neuberg DS, Wain JC, Lynch TJ, Giovannucci E, Christiani DC. Vitamin D is associated with improved survival in early-stage non-small cell lung cancer patients. *Cancer Epidemiol Biomarkers Prev.* 2005 Oct;14(10):2303-9. PMID: 16214909

Acknowledgments

It takes a village for a full-time practicing physician to write a book on a subject that he is so passionate about. There are so many people that I would like to thank for their support, it would take another book to thank them all.

Many thanks to my friend and attorney, Ken Browning, for introducing me to the wonderful people at Hay House, and for all the help he is giving in this project.

At Hay House, I would especially like to thank Reid Tracy for recognizing from our first conversation what this entire vitamin D project could become. My thanks to Jill Kramer and Lisa Mitchell for their excellent help in editing this book; and to Margarete Nielsen and Jeannie Liberati, who helped guide this project. Also my thanks go to Amy Rose Grigoriou for the beautiful art and design she did for the book. Thanks to the many others at Hay House who helped in so many ways.

A special thanks to Christine Wheeler, whom I could always count on in the birthing of this book. From outlines and articles to a finished manuscript, her clarity of thought and ability to help me bring words to my ideas were invaluable.

I am also very grateful to Judie Harvey who so graciously gave her time and expertise in the final editing process of my book.

Many thanks to my friend Guruka Singh Khalsa for his wonderful editing advice, and to his wife Guruka Kaur Khalsa for her support.

I give thanks to my special friend and brother, Joel Roberts, for his inspiration and encouragement throughout this project.

I am grateful to my spiritual sister, Sardarni Guru Amrit Kaur, for the gifts of insight and understanding that she always gives me.

I extend my appreciation and respect to my dear friend Master Sung Baek for the encouragement, inspiration, and spiritual strength he always gives me.

Many thanks to my incredible friends, Gaya Rafiki and Loretta Sparks, who encouraged me and stood by me as this book was conceived and completed. They were an integral part of the process that led to this book.

A special thank you to James Arthur Ray, who has helped me understand faith, trust, and success.

My thanks go to my entire office staff and my wonderful administrator, Jeannie Sakamoto. Thank you all for keeping the office running and for understanding when I had meetings to go to and being willing to schedule the changes required for that.

I also give thanks to my longtime friend and mentor Jeffrey Bland, Ph.D., for his inspirational teaching of nutritional biochemistry, and his introducing me to the importance of vitamin D many years ago.

My thanks to John Cannell, M.D., for reviewing parts of this book and giving me his valuable comments and recommendations. Also I would like to thank Michael Holick, Ph.D., M.D., for answering my questions along the path of writing this book. My thanks also go to all the many vitamin D researchers who have published their groundbreaking and profound articles upon which this book is based. These include John J. Cannell, M.D.; Cedric F. Garland, Dr. P.H.; Frank C. Garland, Ph.D.; Edward Giovannucci, M.D., Sc.D.; Edward D. Gorham, M.P.H., Ph.D.; William B. Grant, Ph.D.; John Hathcock, Ph.D.; Robert P. Heaney, M.D.; Michael F. Holick, Ph.D., M.D.; Bruce W. Hollis, Ph.D.; Joan M. Lappe, Ph.D., R.N.; Anthony W. Norman, Ph.D.; Reinhold Vieth, Ph.D.; and Walter C. Willett, Dr. P.H., M.D.

My thanks to Tej Kaur Khalsa for all the transcribing of my long dictations, and to my friend Seva Kaur Khalsa for her wonderful graphics help.

I give thanks to all my patients who have trusted me and believed in me. On my word, they began to take their "high dose" vitamin D, long before it became the popular thing to do.

All my many personal friends, including Satinder Bhatia, M.D.; Joel Brokaw; Walter Crinnion, N.D.; Harry Levitt; Paul Mittman, N.D.; Shawn Nasseri, M.D.; Alan Schwartz; and Alan Weiss, M.D., who encouraged me as I was writing and were understanding when I canceled dinners and lunches.

Finally, my heart goes out to my saintly wife, Kulwant, who understands me on a deeper level than I even know myself. I give my heartfelt thanks for her encouragement and understanding and her accepting of my time away from our family life.

And most important, I am eternally grateful to my Creator for giving me Guru Ram Das and my spiritual teacher, Yogi Bhajan, to guide my way on.

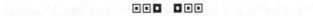

About the Author

Board certified in Internal Medicine, **Soram Khalsa, M.D.**, is a clinical professor of medicine and past chairman of the advisory committee for the Environmental Medicine Center of Excellence at Southwest College of Naturopathic Medicine in Tempe, Arizona. He is also a member of the Bureau of Naturopathic Medicine Advisory Council for the State of California and serves as medical director for the East-West Medical Research Institute. In 2007, Dr. Khalsa was chosen by his peers as one of the "Best Doctors" in America and serves in this capacity as a consultant for integrative medicine.

Dr. Khalsa is a founding member of the American Holistic Medical Association, a founding member of the American Academy of Medical Acupuncture, and was also a member of the Outside Scientific Advisory Board for the NIH-sponsored Center on Botanical Studies at the David Geffen School of Medicine at the University of California, Los Angeles (UCLA). In his private medical practice, he integrates phytotherapeutics, nutrition, homeopathy, acupuncture, and environmental medicine with traditional Internal Medicine.

Dr. Khalsa graduated from Yale University and attended Case Western Reserve School of Medicine in Cleveland. After an internship at St. Luke's Hospital in Cleveland, he completed a residency at the Hospital of the Good Samaritan in Los Angeles. He continued his study of complementary medicine in North America, as well as in Europe and Asia.

Dr. Khalsa is on the medical staff at Cedars-Sinai Medical Center in Los Angeles, California.

In his personal life, Dr Khalsa is a member of the Board of Directors of Sikh Dharma International. He keeps fit with his hobbies of a regular yoga practice for over 35 years, a love of walking, and an enjoyment of dancing.

We hope you enjoyed this Hay House book.
If you'd like to receive our online catalog featuring additional
information on Hay House books and products, or if you'd like to
find out more about the Hay Foundation, please contact:

Hay House, Inc.
P.O. Box 5100
Carlsbad, CA 92018-5100

(760) 431-7695 or **(800) 654-5126**
(760) 431-6948 (fax) or **(800) 650-5115 (fax)**
www.hayhouse.com® • **www.hayfoundation.org**

▣ ▪ ▣

Published and distributed in Australia by: Hay House Australia
Pty. Ltd., 18/36 Ralph St., Alexandria NSW 2015 • *Phone:* 612-9669-
4299 • *Fax:* 612-9669-4144 • www.hayhouse.com.au

Published and distributed in the United Kingdom by: Hay House
UK, Ltd., 292B Kensal Rd., London W10 5BE • *Phone:* 44-20-8962-
1230 • *Fax:* 44-20-8962-1239 • www.hayhouse.co.uk

Published and distributed in the Republic of South Africa by: Hay
House SA (Pty), Ltd., P.O. Box 990, Witkoppen 2068 • *Phone/Fax:*
27-11-467-8904 • info@hayhouse.co.za • www.hayhouse.co.za

Published in India by: Hay House Publishers India, Muskaan
Complex, Plot No. 3, B-2, Vasant Kunj, New Delhi 110 070 • *Phone:*
91-11-4176-1620 • *Fax:* 91-11-4176-1630 • www.hayhouse.co.in

Distributed in Canada by: Raincoast, 9050 Shaughnessy St.,
Vancouver, B.C. V6P 6E5 • *Phone:* (604) 323-7100
Fax: (604) 323-2600 • www.raincoast.com

JOIN THE HAY HOUSE FAMILY

As the leading self-help, mind, body and spirit publisher in the UK, we'd like to welcome you to our family so that you can enjoy all the benefits our website has to offer.

 EXTRACTS from a selection of your favourite author titles

 COMPETITIONS, PRIZES & SPECIAL OFFERS Win extracts, money off, downloads and so much more

 LISTEN to a range of radio interviews and our latest audio publications

 CELEBRATE YOUR BIRTHDAY An inspiring gift will be sent your way

 LATEST NEWS Keep up with the latest news from and about our authors

 ATTEND OUR AUTHOR EVENTS Be the first to hear about our author events

 iPHONE APPS Download your favourite app for your iPhone

 HAY HOUSE INFORMATION Ask us anything, all enquiries answered

join us online at **www.hayhouse.co.uk**

 292B Kensal Road, London W10 5BE
T: 020 8962 1230 E: info@hayhouse.co.uk